Telephone Quitlines

A Resource for Development, Implementation, and Evaluation

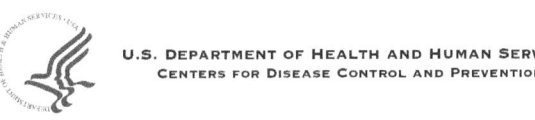
U.S. DEPARTMENT OF HEALTH AND HUMAN SERVICES
CENTERS FOR DISEASE CONTROL AND PREVENTION

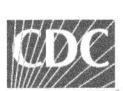

Ordering Information

To order a copy of this publication, contact the

Centers for Disease Control and Prevention
Office on Smoking and Health
Mail Stop K-50, Publications
4770 Buford Highway, NE
Atlanta, GA 30341-3717

Phone: 1-800-CDC-1311 (800-232-1311)
FAX Information Service: 1-888-CDC-FAXX (888-232-3299)

http://www.cdc.gov/tobacco/pubs.htm

Suggested Citation

Centers for Disease Control and Prevention. *Telephone Quitlines: A Resource for Development, Implementation, and Evaluation.* Atlanta, GA: U.S. Department of Health and Human Services, Centers for Disease Control and Prevention, National Center for Chronic Disease Prevention and Health Promotion, Office on Smoking and Health, Final Edition, September 2004.

Table of Contents

Preface v

Acknowledgments vi

1. The Role of Quitlines in Comprehensive Tobacco Control Programs 1
   Efficacy, accessibility, efficiency, interaction with other program components

2. The Range of Practice 9
   Populations served, types of service provided, utilization

3. Contracting for Quitline Services 23
   The request for proposals, selecting a contractor, monitoring the contract

4. Technological Considerations 33
   Telephone systems, information systems

5. Staffing a Quitline 39
   Qualifications needed, staffing levels, training, scheduling, supervision

6. Quality Assurance in Quitline Counseling 47
   Strategies and measures, quality improvement

7. Evaluating a Quitline 53
   The evaluation plan, assessing contributions to the overall tobacco control program, logistical issues

8. Costs Associated with Operating a Quitline 65
   Internal structure of the budget, costs in relation to other tobacco control program activities

9. Promoting Quitlines 71
   The media contractor, traditional and social marketing, channels for promotion, evaluating the campaign

10. Quitline Partnerships 81
    Promotional and referral relationships, integration with the tobacco control program, systems-level partnerships

11. Future Directions 89
    Increasing the menu of services, population impact, partnering for growth, a quitline consortium

References 95

Appendix A: State Quitline Information 103

Appendix B: Vendors Providing Quitline Services to States 107

Appendix C: Cessation Web Resources 109

Appendix D: Client Education Materials Commonly Distributed by Quitlines. 111

Appendix E: Sample Technical Review Instrument 113

Appendix F: Proposed Minimal Data Set for Evaluation of Telephone
Cessation Helplines/Quitlines 117

Appendix G: Health Insurance Portability and Accountability Act (HIPAA) Information . . . 123

Appendix H: Sample Fax Referral Form 125

Appendix I. *Tobacco Quitlines* Fact Sheet. 127

Preface

This document was prepared by the U.S. Department of Health and Human Services under the direction of the Centers for Disease Control and Prevention, National Center for Chronic Disease Prevention and Health Promotion, Office on Smoking and Health, in response to a growing interest in telephone-based tobacco cessation services commonly known as quitlines. It is intended to help state health departments, health care organizations, and employers to contract for and monitor telephone-based tobacco cessation services. It is also intended to help states, health care organizations, and quitline operators enhance existing quitline services, and to inform those who are interested in learning more about population-based approaches to tobacco cessation.

The scientific literature contains little information about contracting for and operating quitline services. The information and recommendations presented in this document are therefore based primarily on the expert opinions of a panel of tobacco control professionals who have experience with statewide quitlines.

Acknowledgments

The Quitline Resource Guide was prepared by the U.S. Department of Health and Human Services under the general editorship of the following individuals from the Centers for Disease Control and Prevention, National Center for Chronic Disease Prevention and Health Promotion, Office on Smoking and Health.

Corinne G. Husten, M.D., M.P.H., Chief, Epidemiology Branch

Abby C. Rosenthal, M.P.H., Cessation Strategic Coordinator

The Centers for Disease Control and Prevention, Office on Smoking and Health, thanks the following individuals for contributing to the preparation of this publication.

Scientific Editor

Shu-Hong Zhu, Ph.D.
Associate Professor
Dept. of Family and Preventive Medicine
University of California, San Diego
La Jolla, CA

Lead Writer

Christopher M. Anderson, B.A.
Program Director
California Smokers' Helpline
Dept. of Family and Preventive Medicine
University of California, San Diego
La Jolla, CA

Contributors

Laura Buss, B.A.
Communications Coordinator
MMSI, a Mayo Health Company
Rochester, MN

Michael Cummings, Ph.D., M.P.H.
Chairman
Cancer Prevention, Epidemiology and Biostatistics
Roswell Park Cancer Institute
Buffalo, NY

Karen Krueger, R.N., M.S.N.
Public Health Nurse Consultant
Tobacco Prevention and Control
Washington State Department of Health
Olympia, WA

K. Joanne Pike, M.A., L.P.C.
Quitline Counseling Manager
American Cancer Society
Austin, TX

Pamela Powers, M.P.H.
Program Director
Network for Information and Counseling
University of Arizona
Tucson, AZ

Sara Tifft, M.B.A.
Marketing Manager
Tobacco Cessation Services
Center for Health Promotion, Inc.
Tukwila, WA

Donna Warner, M.B.A., M.A., C.A.C.
Director, Planning and Program Development
Massachusetts Tobacco Control Program
Massachusetts Department of Public Health
Boston, MA

Reviewers

Dawn Wiesenberger, M.P.H.
Chief, Division of Federal and Special
 Tobacco Control Initiatives
Maryland Department of Health and
 Mental Hygiene
Baltimore, MD

Tim McAfee, M.D., M.P.H.
Chief Medical Officer
Center for Health Promotion, Inc.
Tukwila, WA

Paul McDonald, Ph.D.
Associate Professor
Department of Health Studies
University of Waterloo
Waterloo, Ontario
Canada

Clarysse Nunokawa, M.S.W.
Program Officer
Hawaii Community Foundation
Honolulu, HI

Melva Fager Okun, Dr.P.H.
Facilitator
North Carolina Prevention Partners
University of North Carolina
Institute of Public Health
Chapel Hill, NC

Deborah Ossip-Klein, Ph.D.
Chief, Social and Behavioral Medicine
James P. Wilmot Cancer Center
University of Rochester School of Medicine
Rochester, NY

Karen Siener, M.P.H.
Program Consultant
Office on Smoking and Health
Centers for Disease Control and Prevention
Atlanta, GA

Margy Wienbar, M.S.
Quality Improvement Manager
New Mexico Medical Review Association
Albuquerque, NM

Eileen Yam
North Carolina Prevention Partners Intern
University of North Carolina
Institute of Public Health
Chapel Hill, NC

Staff

Jody Gan, M.P.H., C.H.E.S.
Senior Technical Assistance Specialist
Northrop Grumman Information
 Technology Health Solutions
Rockville, MD

Maxine Forrest, B.A.
Senior Technical Writer
Northrop Grumman Information
 Technology Health Solutions
Rockville, MD

The Role of Quitlines in Comprehensive Tobacco Control Programs

Overview

Tobacco use continues to be the leading cause of death and disease in the United States; more than 440,000 people in this country die of tobacco-related diseases each year (CDC 2002a). Fortunately, cessation of tobacco use can reduce the risk of tobacco-related disease, even among those who have used tobacco for decades (USDHHS 2000a, USDHHS 2000b, Peto et al. 2000, Taylor et al. 2002). Cessation also saves money; tobacco use is estimated to cost the nation close to $157 billion annually in excess medical expenses and lost productivity (CDC 2002a).

Cessation rates, however, have been low. One recent national survey indicates that about 41% of smokers try to quit smoking each year, but only 4.7% maintain abstinence for at least 3 months (CDC 2002b).

An increase in either the percentage of tobacco users making quit attempts or in the success rate for such attempts can lead to a higher overall cessation rate (Burns 2000). Traditional cessation programs have mostly focused on the latter, assisting those who are trying to quit and actively seek help in doing so. They have not often sought to increase the rate of quit attempts in the general population. In other words, traditional cessation programs have adopted a clinical rather than a public health approach (Lichtenstein & Glasgow 1992). Over the past decade, however, there has been an effort to adopt a more public health-oriented approach to cessation (Niaura & Abrams 2002), that is, one that is concerned not only with the cessation rate of the individuals who seek help to quit, but with that of all tobacco users in the population. In this approach, cessation becomes an integral part of a comprehensive tobacco control program, by making help available for those who seek it, and by actively promoting cessation in the general population.

> An increase either in the percentage of tobacco users making quit attempts or in the success rate for those attempts can lead to a higher overall cessation rate.

The Role of Quitlines in Comprehensive Tobacco Control Programs

Telephone-based tobacco cessation services, commonly known as quitlines, have shown the potential to address both of these aims. First, their effectiveness with smokers who use them is well established (Hopkins et al. 2001, Lichtenstein et al. 1996, Stead et al. 2004). Second, in many states with comprehensive tobacco control programs, quitlines play an integral role in media-based efforts to increase quit attempts in the general population (Zhu 2000). Consequently, as of 2003, 40 states have established some form of quitline (CDC unpublished data). This chapter briefly discusses the reasons quitlines are well suited to lead the cessation component of a comprehensive tobacco control program.

Quitlines Are Effective in Helping Tobacco Users Quit

Several meta-analytic reviews have established that proactive telephone counseling is an effective intervention for smoking cessation (Lichtenstein et al. 1996, Fiore et al. 2000, Hopkins et al. 2001, Stead et al. 2004). The current U.S. Public Health Clinical Practice Guideline and the Guide to Community Preventive Services both recommend proactive telephone counseling as a method to help smokers quit (Fiore et al. 2000, Hopkins et al. 2001).

Proactive Quitlines

Most of the quitline studies conducted so far have focused on proactive quitlines. Proactive quitlines may provide some form of immediate "reactive" assistance when a tobacco user first calls, but they also provide more comprehensive services through outbound ("proactive") calls. The outbound service, which often entails multiple follow-up sessions, is typically scheduled by agreement with the smoker. Randomized, controlled trials have established the efficacy of such proactive interventions, with the most recent meta-analysis of 13 studies showing a 56% increase in quit rates when compared with self-help (Stead et al. 2004).

Several of these quitline studies were conducted under real-world or near real-world conditions, making application of the findings fairly straightforward (Lichtenstein et al. 2003). Proven treatments sometimes fail in practice because translation from clinical trials to service settings may involve changes in the conditions under which the original results were obtained (Flay 1986, Greenwald & Cullen 1985, Stevens et al. 2000). The effectiveness of quitlines, however, has been demonstrated in the context of existing quitline service operations, and in fact quitlines have been shown to provide a robust behavioral service for people who want to quit smoking (Borland et al. 2001, Zhu et al. 2002).

Reactive Quitlines

Reactive quitlines, which respond to callers' immediate requests for assistance but do not provide outbound counseling calls, have not been studied as widely as proactive quitlines. Although there is some evidence of its effectiveness, this strategy has not been recommended by the various guidelines.

There are two studies in the literature that support the use of reactive quitlines in the context of comprehensive tobacco control programs. In one study, a well-promoted quitline that provided a single, yet substantial (50-minute), pre-quit counseling session to smokers was shown to increase callers' quit attempts and reduce the incidence of relapse, when compared with an intervention that provided callers with only self-help materials (Zhu et al. 1996). In another study, communities in which a quitline was promoted were shown to have significantly higher quit attempt rates and significantly higher overall cessation rates than similar communities without a promoted quitline. This was true despite the fact that only a minority of smokers with access to the quitline actually called (Ossip-Klein et al. 1991). It is unclear whether the increase in cessation was the result of promotion alone or promotion in conjunction with the quitline itself. Media campaigns in conjunction with a variety of community interventions have been shown to increase cessation (Hopkins et al. 2001). A possible explanation for this phenomenon is that knowledge of cessation services, engendered through promotion, increases tobacco users' belief in the normalcy of quitting, which may lead to increased quit attempts among people who have access to the services, even those who do not use them. In other words, promotion of a quitline in itself may lead to additional quit attempts, which may in turn lead to greater permanent quitting success in the communities where it is promoted (Zhu 2000). More studies are needed to assess the efficacy of reactive quitlines. In the meantime, it is clear that states with reactive quitlines should spend significant resources on promotion (Wakefield & Borland 2000).

Most existing statewide quitlines have employed both proactive and reactive elements (Ossip-Klein & McIntosh 2003). The overall evidence indicates that such quitlines have the potential not only to provide effective assistance to those who seek it but also to increase quitting among tobacco users generally. Existing quitline budgets are sometimes insufficient to provide full service to all who want to use

> Quitlines have been shown to provide a robust behavioral service for people who want to quit smoking.

> The overall evidence indicates that quitlines have the potential not only to provide effective assistance to those who seek it but also to increase quitting among tobacco users generally.

them, and there is ongoing discussion among quitline operators about what is the best distribution of their efforts and which populations are best served within these budget constraints (Zhu 2002a).

Quitlines Are Accessible and Efficient

Aside from their proven effectiveness, quitlines have other advantages that have made them a top cessation strategy for states. These advantages have led the Interagency Committee on Smoking and Health, Cessation Subcommittee, to recommend the establishment of a national network of state-managed quitlines to provide universal coverage for tobacco cessation (Fiore et al. 2004).

One important advantage of quitlines is their accessibility. A telephone operation eliminates many of the barriers of traditional cessation classes, such as having to wait for classes to form or needing to arrange for transportation. Quitlines are particularly helpful for people with limited mobility and those who live in rural or remote areas. Due to their quasi-anonymous nature, telephonic services may also appeal to those who are reluctant to seek help provided in a group setting, helping them overcome what can be a significant psychological barrier (Zhu & Anderson 2000). As evidence of the greater accessibility of quitlines, surveys have indicated that smokers are several times more likely to use such a service than they are to use a face-to-face program (McAfee et al. 1998, Zhu & Anderson 2000). In fact, quitlines have little trouble keeping their counselors busy as thousands of tobacco users call for help (Owen 2000, Wakefield and Borland 2000, and Zhu et al. 2000). Moreover, populations that are underrepresented in traditional cessation services, such as smokers of ethnic minority backgrounds, actively seek help from quitlines (Zhu et al. 1995).

Another advantage of quitlines is that the centralized nature of their operations creates opportunities for efficiency in executing the cessation component of a state's tobacco control program. A single large-scale promotional campaign for a statewide quitline is more feasible than numerous smaller campaigns for a wide range of local programs. A centralized quitline can also serve as an information clearinghouse and provide direct referrals to local programs for callers who want to use them. Centralization of counseling services brings an economy of scale. Since demand for quitline services is largely a function of how much they are promoted, which is itself a controllable factor, it is possible to staff a quitline so that all staff members are efficiently utilized. This is not always the case with smaller local programs that are more vulnerable to fluctuating

> Populations that are underrepresented in traditional cessation services, such as smokers of ethnic minority backgrounds, actively seek help from quitlines.

demand. In fact, the economy of scale may be sufficient to enable the quitline to offer multilingual and other specialized services to users, which would be cost-prohibitive for most local cessation clinics. The economy of scale associated with a centralized operation is the main reason that many states consider a quitline to be the primary strategy in a statewide cessation program: It acts as a safety net for the great majority of tobacco users statewide, a consideration that is even more important when states suffer cuts in their cessation budgets.

Interaction with Other Elements of a Comprehensive Tobacco Control Program

A comprehensive tobacco control program typically has four major goals (CDC 1999):

- ◆ Prevent initiation
- ◆ Increase cessation
- ◆ Reduce exposure to secondhand smoke
- ◆ Eliminate disparities in tobacco use and access to treatment

Quitlines focus on cessation, but other components of a comprehensive program also promote quitting, even if they do not directly provide cessation services. Media campaigns are an obvious example, but there are others. A health care system that has been mobilized to increase physician advice to smokers also promotes quitting. School-based programs, while focusing on prevention, may promote quitting among adolescent smokers. Work site restrictions on smoking and efforts to increase tobacco taxes or raise the unit price promote quitting as well (Burns 2000, Hopkins et al. 2001).

Secondhand smoke policies and price increases for tobacco products create pressure on tobacco users to quit, without necessarily providing any help to do so. If cessation services are not available, this pressure runs the risk of appearing punitive to tobacco users. However, this risk is lessened in states with well-promoted and widely available cessation services. As a single centralized operation with recognizable branding and universal toll-free access, a quitline is a good way to let tobacco users, wherever they are, know that help is available if they need it. In this way, a quitline complements other tobacco control activities that increase tobacco users' desire to quit. Such interactions create a synergy among different components of the program (Burns 2000).

The Role of Quitlines in Comprehensive Tobacco Control Programs

> Secondhand smoke ads, ostensibly focused on protecting the health of nonsmokers, became an efficient way to encourage smokers to use a cessation service.

This synergy can be seen most clearly in the collaboration between a state's quitline and its media campaign (see Chapter 9). The media have been used extensively to educate the public about the dangers of smoking, and a common theme of such campaigns is the harmfulness of secondhand smoke (Stevens 1998). This theme is only indirectly related to cessation, but the two themes can be linked. For example, through a careful creative process, California's media campaign developed secondhand smoke ads that also promoted the quitline. Because the quitline's number was included, the cessation message in the ads became more complete, not only providing smokers with a reason to quit but also offering them help to do so. Interestingly, the secondhand smoke ads outperformed basic health ads in generating calls to the quitline. Thus, secondhand smoke ads, ostensibly focused on protecting the health of nonsmokers, became an efficient way to encourage smokers to use a cessation service (Anderson & Zhu 2000).

Another potential area for synergy among program components is to use quitlines to support physician advice to quit smoking (see Chapter 10). The U.S. Public Health Service guideline recommends that physicians ask about their patients' smoking status at every visit, advise every smoker to quit, and prescribe or recommend Food and Drug Administration-approved medications for every quit attempt in the absence of major medical contraindications. The guideline further suggests that physicians should help their patients formulate a quit plan, provide supplementary materials, and schedule a follow-up session to be conducted either in person or via the telephone (Fiore et al. 2000). In practice, time constraints and a lack of training on how to counsel their patients on cessation create barriers to physician implementation of the guideline. What physicians can easily do, however, is screen for tobacco use, advise tobacco users to quit, and refer patients to the quitline for cessation counseling (Schroeder 2003).

Collaboration between a quitline and other components of a comprehensive tobacco control program can also help eliminate disparities between various populations with respect to tobacco use and its toll on health and access to effective treatment services. For example, people of ethnic minority backgrounds are collectively less likely to use cessation services than whites (USDHHS 1998). In some cases, language can be a barrier to access. As mentioned previously, it would be cost-prohibitive to ensure that all local cessation programs across a state had multilingual capabilities. It is more feasible to address such a disparity in a centralized operation where separate language lines can be set up to cover the entire state or region. A media campaign using actors from the target community and conducted in the target language can both promote cessation in that community and encourage its members to access available services, thereby helping to address the disparity of access. Data from California have shown that a culturally and linguistically targeted campaign that is tagged with a quitline number can draw smokers of ethnic minority backgrounds as effectively as the general market campaign draws white smokers (Zhu et al. 1995). In this case, quitlines help address disparities by providing a "level playing field" in access to service.

The Range of Practice

Overview

All quitlines in the United States provide some sort of individual cessation assistance, but they vary significantly in several important ways. They employ different combinations of service modalities and range considerably in the size and scope of their operations. The populations they serve vary with respect to readiness to quit and cultural and linguistic backgrounds. Quitlines also vary in addressing specific populations such as tobacco users from low-income households, pregnant women, adolescents, and users of smokeless tobacco products, such as chewing tobacco.

This chapter explores and contrasts the various statewide quitline services offered in the United States. The goal is to document the current range of practice and to identify important considerations for those who fund or operate quitlines and those who are preparing to do so. Included at the end of the chapter is a case study highlighting services provided by the California Smokers' Helpline—the nation's oldest statewide quitline.

Populations Served

Readiness to Quit

Telephone counseling has been seen primarily as a means of helping tobacco users quit and only secondarily as a means of moving tobacco users along the continuum of readiness to quit. Most research trials demonstrating the efficacy of proactive telephone counseling for smoking cessation have served callers who were almost ready to quit when they made their first call. Most quitlines still spend the bulk of their resources on such callers. In fact, several quitlines reserve counseling, their most intensive and expensive service, for those who report that they are ready to make a quit attempt; many others require a commitment to quit within a certain timeframe. For example, California offers counseling services for those ready to quit

> Several quitlines reserve counseling, their most expensive service, for those ready to make a quit attempt.

The Range of Practice

within a week, and Arizona reserves counseling for those ready to quit within 30 days. Both states, however, send motivational materials to callers who do not yet fit these descriptions and invite them to call back for counseling when they do.

Some programs also target tobacco users who are not yet ready to quit. For example, Blue Cross Blue Shield of Minnesota established a private quitline for its members that actively recruits callers at all stages of readiness. Funders of statewide, public quitlines must also consider whether they will offer counseling to those who are not ready to quit in the near future. There is some evidence that telephone counseling can benefit even those who, at baseline, are not planning to quit (Curry et al. 1995).

Cultural and Linguistic Diversity

Statewide quitlines serve English-speakers of all races and backgrounds, and most of them also provide services in Spanish. Some quitlines advertise only in English and Spanish, but retain staff members who speak other languages and use their language skills when needed. Other quitlines use third-party translation services, such as AT&T Interpretive Services, to increase the number of languages supported.

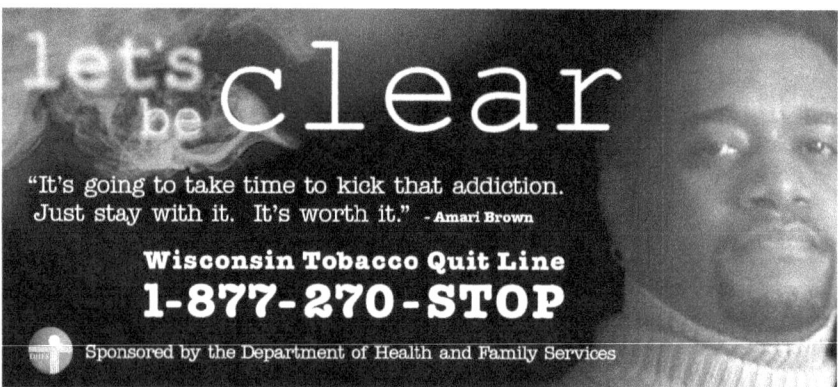

Wisconsin Tobacco Control Board 2003. "Let's Be Clear" media campaign ad targeting African American smokers.

Quitlines serving regions with ethnic minority populations must carefully consider the cultural and linguistic appropriateness of their programs. An ethnically and linguistically diverse base of callers presents a wide range of expectations for service, and all elements of the quitline, from outreach and promotion to programming and staff training, must address this range of expectations. For example, a service successfully billed as "counseling" in English-speaking communities may fare better if billed as "help" or "information" in Asian-language communities, where use of programs perceived as mental health services is often stigmatized.

Studies to establish the efficacy of proactive telephone counseling for smoking cessation have included English- and Spanish-speaking participants of ethnically diverse backgrounds, but no significant differences in outcomes along ethnic or linguistic lines have been reported, suggesting that this type of counseling may be effective for English- and Spanish-speaking smokers from many racial and ethnic backgrounds (Stead et al. 2004). As yet, the field has not established an evidence base for Asian-language quitlines.

Low-Income Tobacco Users

Quitlines may receive many calls from tobacco users with low socioeconomic status (SES) (Anderson & Zhu 2002). Quitlines should make special efforts to reach this segment of the population, which has the highest prevalence of tobacco use of any socioeconomic group (USDHHS 2000b). If resources are insufficient to provide comprehensive services to all callers who want them, states may consider prioritizing low-SES tobacco users to help address this disparity.

> States may consider prioritizing low-SES tobacco users to help address the disparity in prevalence.

Studies establishing the efficacy of proactive telephone counseling for smoking cessation have included participants of diverse socioeconomic backgrounds, but no significant differences in outcomes along socioeconomic lines have been reported, suggesting that low-SES tobacco users can benefit from evidence-based counseling protocols.

Pregnant Smokers

Quitline media campaigns aimed at the general population of adult smokers generate a significant number of calls from pregnant smokers. Many quitlines have responded to this demand by developing special protocols addressing the unique needs of pregnant smokers, and studies testing the effectiveness of these protocols have begun to show promising results (Cummins et al. 2002). In addition, the scientific literature for other counseling venues provides some guidance in the development of specialized protocols for pregnant smokers (Melvin et al. 2000). Because smoking while pregnant is more common among women of low SES, such protocols must address the increased social and economic instability in which many pregnant smokers live, relative to the general smoking population. These circumstances may make it more difficult for the quitline to reach pregnant women for proactive counseling. Another challenge is the

The Range of Practice

> Most quitlines actively assist pregnant callers given the potential danger of smoking to fetal health.

high rate of postpartum relapse: as many as 70% of women who quit during pregnancy return to smoking within 6 months after delivery (Floyd 1993).

Despite these challenges, most quitlines actively assist pregnant callers given the potential danger of smoking to fetal health. National organizations have become involved in the effort as well. Smoke-Free Families is a multisite, multiphase, biobehavioral research program that is exploring innovative approaches to prevent smoking during pregnancy and beyond (Orleans et al. 2004). Great Start is a national media campaign that encourages women to call the Great Start quitline service, jointly sponsored by the American Legacy Foundation and the American Cancer Society. Given the recent increase in cessation efforts directed at this population, states and quitline operators should monitor the scientific literature for developments relating to telephone interventions for pregnant smokers.

Adolescent Smokers

Media campaigns to promote quitlines generate calls from tobacco users of all ages, including adolescents. In response, many U.S. quitlines have developed specialized protocols for underage smokers. While the proportion of quitline callers who are younger than 18 is small (less than 2% in 2001) (Zhu 2002a), they often receive considerable attention from quitline funders and operators. Interest in this population is high because studies have shown that most long-term smokers start smoking as teenagers. Another concern is that in most areas, very few teen cessation services are available.

The main challenge encountered by states that want to provide quitlines for teens is the lack of proven models for long-term effective interventions with adolescent tobacco users. Teens have not been included as participants in most of the major trials of quitline efficacy (Zhu 2002b). Another challenge is that in addition to the relapse pressures that ex-smokers of all ages face (uncomfortable withdrawal symptoms, for example), adolescent ex-smokers may also face "reuptake" pressures (Zhu 2003). These include the influence of aggressive, age-specific marketing by the tobacco industry and social pressure from peers who may regard smoking as socially desirable. A third challenge is the requirement in many states that quitline staff obtain parental consent before providing proactive counseling to teenage callers. This requirement decreases the likelihood of teens receiving the intended service, not so much because teens are afraid their parents or guardians will discover they smoke (they usually already know), but because contacting the parents or guardians and then recontacting the teens can be logistically difficult (Zhu 2003).

Despite these challenges, most quitlines offer at least a minimal level of service to teens who call. However, until the evidence base has been more firmly established, it is not recommended that states aggressively promote services for this population (Zhu 2003). Funders and quitline operators should monitor the scientific literature for developments in this area. Recent cessation efforts with teens have met with modest success, so there is reason to be cautiously optimistic (Hollis et al. 2002, Zhu 2003, McDonald et al. 2003, Mermelstein 2003).

> It is not recommended that quitlines aggressively promote services for teens until the evidence base has been more firmly established.

Chewing Tobacco Users

The use of chewing tobacco is a serious public health concern, especially in rural areas (CDC 1993b). Quitline media campaigns, even if they do not specifically target this audience, result in small but significant numbers of calls from "chewers." In response, most quitlines have developed special protocols for working with them (Zhu 2002a).

Quitline operators may find that callers who chew are more likely than callers who smoke to be young, white, and male (Padgett et al. 2002). Because the great majority of anti-tobacco messages have focused on smoking, chewers may have less knowledge about the health risks of chewing tobacco than smokers have about the risks of smoking. Chewers also have different triggers and absorb nicotine differently than smokers do. For this reason, some quitting strategies that work well for smokers may be less effective for chewers (Hatsukami & Severson 1999).

While quitlines for smoking cessation have been more widely studied and proven effective, there is also evidence that telephone counseling can be effective for chewing tobacco cessation (Severson et al. 2000). Mass media promotion of chewing tobacco quitline services may be less cost-efficient, however, since chewers comprise a much smaller portion of the general population than smokers and are less likely to live in urban areas where most media campaigns are aired. The extent to which states dedicate resources to treating the use of chewing tobacco should be guided by statewide assessments of chewing tobacco usage and its toll on public health.

Types of Service Provided

Counseling

All quitlines provide some sort of counseling intervention, but there is considerable variety in how the counseling is provided, particularly with regard to intensity. Quitlines can design their counseling intensity

The Range of Practice

> Some states, such as Illinois and New York, provide brief, on-the-spot, one-time counseling to all smokers who call during operating hours.

to be consistent with their mission. They may provide a basic level of service to the greatest number of callers, or a maximally effective time-intensive service to a more limited number of callers, or a mixture of both strategies.

The quitlines of some states, such as Illinois and New York, operate on a reactive, hotline basis, providing brief, on-the-spot, one-time counseling to smokers who call during operating hours. This approach allows a quitline to provide minimal counseling services to a large number of callers.

Many other states offer more time-intensive, proactive counseling that may begin with a reactive session when a tobacco user first calls the quitline. For example, Arizona provides a comprehensive planning session that lasts a little over half an hour. The caller then has a choice of continuing with proactive counseling (for up to eight sessions), receiving a referral to a local group counseling program, or both. Some states triage callers, providing reactive support to all callers and proactive follow-up only to the uninsured or other priority populations.

Some states with relatively large quitlines augment the counseling staff with a group of intake specialists. These specialists answer the majority of incoming calls and collect basic demographic, personal, and behavioral information, explain available services, and record each caller's choice of services. Callers who want counseling may be directly transferred to an available counselor, scheduled for an appointment at a time that is convenient for them, or told that a counselor will be contacting them within the next couple of days.

> Other states offer more time-intensive, proactive counseling. Arizona provides a comprehensive planning session that lasts a little over half an hour.

Quitlines that provide proactive follow-up sessions differ in the scheduling of calls. California's quitline schedules follow-up sessions according to the probability of relapse, with the first call occurring within 24 hours of quitting and subsequent calls at 3 days, 1 week, 2 weeks, and 1 month. Thus, the sessions are "front-loaded" around the quit day and become less frequent as the probability of relapse diminishes. In most cases, all sessions are concluded within a month of the quit date. This model has the advantage of preventing relapse before it happens or addressing it soon afterward (Zhu et al. 1996). In some states, the Free & Clear program provided by the Center for Health Promotion offers a similar number of follow-up sessions, with the first session scheduled shortly after the quit date and the other sessions distributed over a 3- to 4-month period, at the rate of one session per month. This model has the advantage of identifying callers who have relapsed and creating an opportunity to encourage them to quit again (Orleans et al. 1991).

The Range of Practice

Pharmacotherapy

Many quitlines help eligible callers obtain pharmacotherapeutic quitting aids such as nicotine replacement therapy (NRT) or bupropion (Zyban®) (Waa et al. 2000). California provides a certificate of enrollment in quitline services, which, together with a prescription from their doctor, enables callers who are insured by Medicaid to obtain free nicotine patches, nicotine gum, or bupropion at their local pharmacy. Some other insurance plans also honor these certificates. Maine, Minnesota, Utah and Washington State provide NRT directly to eligible callers who participate in comprehensive, proactive counseling. Because the efficacy of NRT and bupropion was demonstrated in trials that usually involved counseling support (Fiore et al. 2000), it is appropriate that quitlines play a role in facilitating smokers' use of these medications (Swan et al. 2003).

Many NRT products, including the patch, gum, and lozenge, have been approved by the Food and Drug Administration for over-the-counter sales, and thus there are few medical or legal concerns about quitlines providing these products. Some private quitlines even dispense bupropion and prescription forms of NRT (e.g., the nasal spray and inhaler). They have developed mechanisms to inform the caller's provider of the recommendation prior to mailing the medication to the client, to ensure concurrence with the prescription.

Referral

Most quitlines maintain updated listings of local cessation programs to which they refer callers who want face-to-face counseling or group support. In an innovative statewide cessation project called QuitWorks, Massachusetts helps callers enroll in local programs. Some quitlines transfer callers directly to their health plans if those plans provide counseling or other cessation benefits such as NRT or bupropion. Most quitlines also have procedures for identifying and referring callers with mental health issues that fall outside the scope of the quitline or that exceed the training of their counselors. Long-time quitline operators have observed the necessity of ensuring that their staff are aware of the most reliable resources for callers in crisis and know when to break confidentiality to ensure safety (for example, to report a suicide threat to the local police or to report suspected child abuse to child protective services).

Mailings

Packets of self-help materials represent one of the least intensive services provided by quitlines, and are usually provided to all callers. The packets may be matched to the caller's level of readiness to quit,

> California, Maine, Massachusetts, Minnesota, Utah and Washington State use various methods to help callers obtain free or reduced-cost nicotine replacement therapy.

> Because the efficacy of NRT and bupropion was demonstrated in trials that also involved counseling, it is appropriate that quitlines play a role in facilitating the use of these medications.

or they may be designed for specific populations, such as chewers, teens, pregnant smokers, and non-English speakers. They may be further customized according to concerns that arise during the first interview (Borland et al. 2004). Arizona, for example, has developed fact sheets covering a wide range of topics, which are selectively included in callers' packets to supplement the basic materials. Some quitlines also enclose smoking substitutes such as a worry stone or a straw.

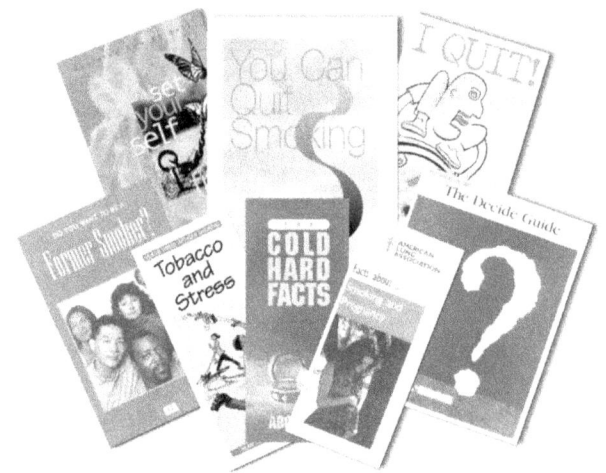

Examples of materials provided by quitlines.

> Self-help materials have not been demonstrated to be efficacious when used on their own, but they provide all callers with at least a basic level of support.

Self-help materials have not been demonstrated to be efficacious when used on their own (Fiore et al. 2000). However, since many quitline callers may be ineligible for counseling services (such as those with private insurance), may not be willing to quit within a specified time period (e.g., 30 days), or may choose not to receive counseling, these relatively inexpensive self-help materials allow quitlines to provide every caller with at least a basic level of support. Self-help materials are also used to supplement any counseling services provided. (See Appendix D for a list of some of the self-help materials provided by quitlines.)

Web Sites

Most state quitlines have a Web site. Some states simply provide an online brochure that directs visitors to the quitline. Others also provide a modest intervention component, and a few states offer comprehensive Web-based cessation services. New Jersey offers both a quitline and Web-based services, and has experienced little overlap between users of the two programs. This state's experience suggests that incorporating Web-based services may be a promising way for other state tobacco control programs to increase their reach. Because there is not yet an evidence base to support Internet interventions, it is not recommended that limited cessation dollars be spent on online services. However, several Web-based cessation programs are currently under evaluation, so states should monitor the scientific literature for developments in this area.

Since Web sites represent a cessation activity distinct from that of quitlines, they are not discussed at length in this document. However, a list of cessation sites currently offered by states is presented in Appendix C.

Utilization of Quitlines

The call volume of new quitlines often undergoes alternating "feast or famine" phases in the first years of operation, until the mechanisms promoting the service are fully understood. Initially, advertising drives utilization, and fluctuations in the level of promotion lead directly to fluctuations in call volume. The first statewide quitline, established by California in 1992, registered more than 14,000 callers during its first 12 months of operation but experienced a large variation in monthly call volume, as shown in Figure 2.1. The peaks in call volume were the direct result of relatively heavy media advertising, while the valleys corresponded to lulls in the campaign. Many other quitlines have experienced similar fluctuations in utilization due to sporadic media promotion. With improvements in coordination between the states, their advertising contractors, and quitline operators, the call volume can become steadier and more predictable over time.

Figure 2.1 California Smokers' Helpline Monthly Call Volume, August 1992–July 1993

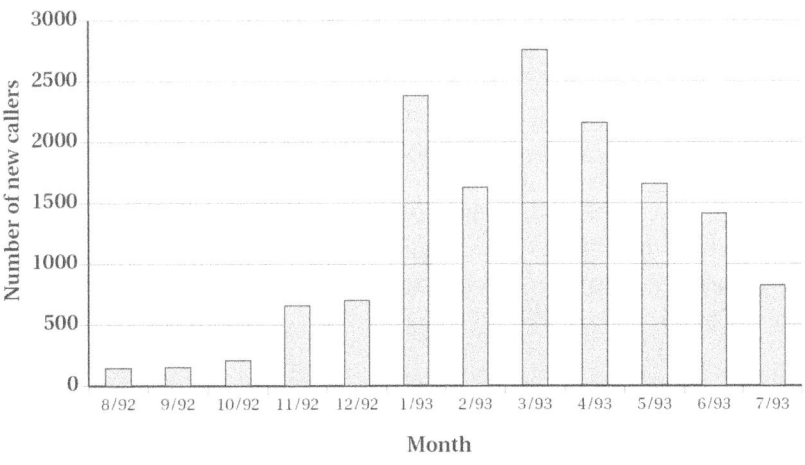

The Range of Practice

> The occasional dramatic spikes in demand following suddenly intensified campaigns suggest that the primary limiting factor in the utilization of quitlines is funding.

Gradually, as a quitline begins to fill gaps in the availability of cessation services and word-of-mouth referrals begin to supplement the media campaign, the quitline may generate greater demand among tobacco users. Figure 2.2, depicting the annual call volume of the California Smokers' Helpline during the first decade of operation, illustrates the steady growth in demand experienced by this quitline. This growth is attributed not only to increased advertising but also to the branding of the quitline and to grassroots efforts to "institutionalize" the service in the minds of people throughout the state who are in a position to refer tobacco users to the quitline. These individuals include doctors, nurses, pharmacists, educators, and others who interact with tobacco users every day.

Figure 2.2 California Smokers' Helpline Annual Call Volume, 1993–2002

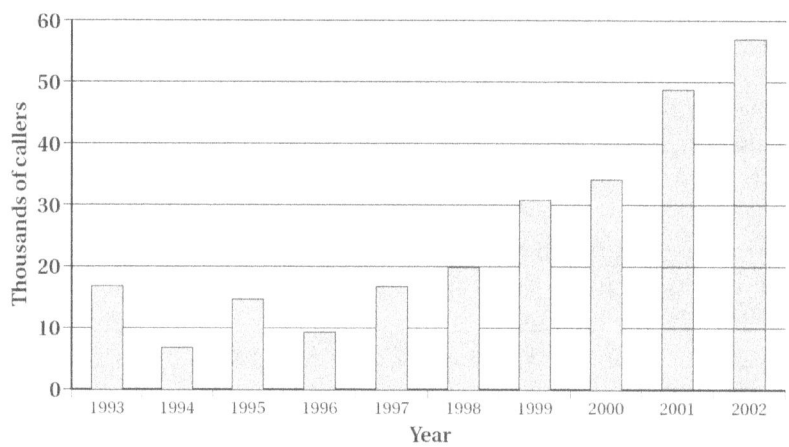

In 2001, 28 statewide quitlines were used by more than 241,000 people, which represents 1% to 5% of the tobacco users in the states that had quitlines. These utilization rates compare very favorably with other cessation programs, but there is still ample room for expansion (McAfee 2002, Zhu 2002a). The occasional dramatic spikes in demand that follow suddenly intensified media campaigns suggest that the primary limiting factor in the utilization of quitlines is funding, both for promotion and for operations.

Figure 2.3 shows the distribution of state quitlines as of January 2004; 38 states and the District of Columbia had active quitlines at that time. (Please see Appendix A for a chart with information about each state quitline.)

Figure 2.3 State Quitlines as of January 2004

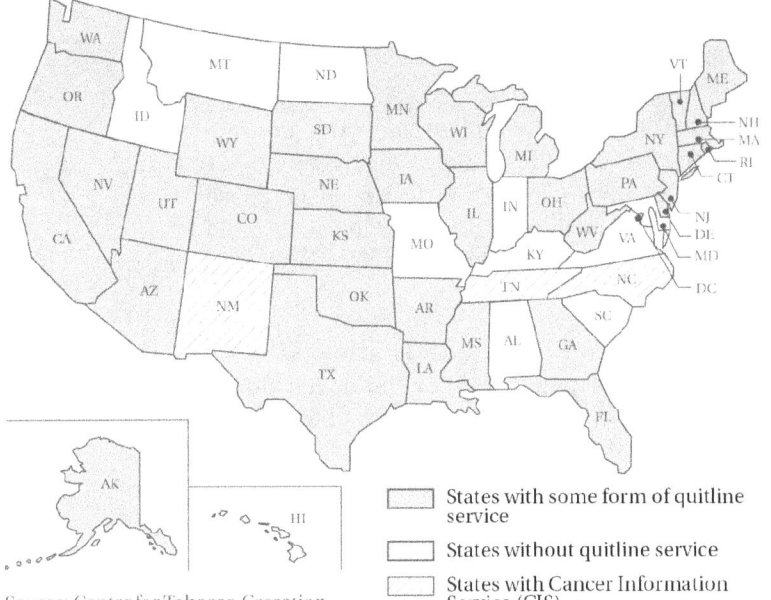

Source: Center for Tobacco Cessation

☐ States with some form of quitline service
☐ States without quitline service
☐ States with Cancer Information Service (CIS)

New Jersey Quitline Reaches Out to the Hispanic/Latino Community

Marta Mangual started smoking with her girlfriends when she was 24 years old and worked her way up to three packs a day by age 67. Although she tried to quit by using nicotine gum, Marta found she could not stay off cigarettes on her own. That changed the day her daughter brought home a brochure for the New Jersey Quitline's Spanish-language service that she had picked up at the supermarket. "After just one call, I felt more motivated than ever," Marta reports. "The counselors were friendly, they seemed to genuinely want to help me, and best of all, I was able to share my feelings about smoking in my native language."

Marta has nothing but great things to say about the quitline. She has been smoke-free for more than a year, and says she thinks it will last this time. "I haven't felt this good in years!" she declares. When asked if she would recommend the Spanish-language service to her friends, Marta quickly replies, "I already have! The New Jersey Quitline es muy bueno!"

(New Jersey Comprehensive Tobacco Control Program 2001)

The Range of Practice

Case Study

Nation's First Statewide Quitline Is Thriving

Since its inception in 1992, the California Smokers' Helpline has served more than 300,000 callers. In 2002 alone, nearly 57,000 callers used the Helpline, which is operated by the University of California, San Diego, and funded through tobacco taxes administered by the California Department of Health Services and the California Children and Families Commission. The Helpline's services include self-help kits, referrals to local programs, and one-on-one telephone counseling.

The state of California has a very diverse population, and the Helpline uses a variety of strategies to reach out to different segments of that population. Services are provided in English, Spanish, Mandarin, Cantonese, Vietnamese, and Korean, and each of these language groups is strongly represented among Helpline callers. Targeted advertising in urban areas and grassroots efforts in rural areas have helped achieve geographic diversity. The state helpline also partnered with the state Medicaid program to help beneficiaries receive pharmacotherapy, which helps to ensure active participation by tobacco users of low socioeconomic status.

Tobacco users calling the Helpline for the first time are asked a brief series of questions assessing tobacco consumption and readiness to quit, as well as contact information and demographics. Callers are then offered a range of Helpline services. At a minimum, they receive a "quit kit" consisting of self-help materials appropriate to their stage of readiness and a descriptive list of cessation resources available in their area.

Callers who choose to receive counseling work with a trained cessation counselor who spends about 40 minutes helping them prepare to quit. The first session covers current tobacco use and quitting history, smoking-related health concerns, social and environmental challenges and resources, planning for difficult situations, and setting a quit date. Counselors use motivational interviewing techniques intended to uncover and enhance callers' inherent motivation for change. They also help callers develop greater confidence in their ability to succeed at quitting.

Subsequent sessions are timed to help prevent relapse, with the most extensive help being provided during the early stages of the quitting process. In the most comprehensive protocol, the counselor follows up within 24 hours of quitting, and again within 3 days, 1 week, 2 weeks, and 1 month. In the beginning, the follow-up sessions focus on immediate concerns such as dealing with withdrawal symptoms, learning from relapse, modifying quitting strategies as needed, and boosting motivation. With time, the focus of the sessions shifts to long-term maintenance issues, such as planning for highly emotional situations and adopting the self-image of a nonsmoker, rather than that of a smoker who is simply not smoking.

The Helpline's counseling service is based on protocols that were proven effective in a large, randomized, controlled trial in San Diego County before implementation of the statewide service (Zhu et al. 1996) and again later in the context of ongoing statewide operations (Zhu et al. 2002). In the original study the effect of multiple proactive counseling sessions was significantly greater than that of a single counseling session, and nearly double that of self-help materials alone (12-month continuous abstinence rates of 26.7%, 19.8%, and 14.7%, respectively).

Recommendations

- Provide a mix of reactive and proactive services to maximize the overall impact of the quitline. As funding permits, expand the provision of proactive counseling, which has the strongest evidence of efficacy.

- Facilitate access to and use of effective pharmacotherapeutic quitting aids such as nicotine patches, nicotine gum, and bupropion.

- Carefully consider the cultural appropriateness of the quitline's services for the populations they are intended to serve. Provide in-language counseling for linguistic minority communities, as feasible.

- Target low-income tobacco users for participation in telephone cessation services, since they have a higher prevalence of tobacco use.

- Provide proactive counseling to help pregnant smokers quit. Recent evidence has shown the efficacy of counseling protocols designed for this population.

- Provide counseling to adolescent smokers, but do not devote a major portion of resources to aggressively promote services for this population until there is a firmer evidence base to support telephone counseling for teen cessation.

- Consider providing counseling for chewing tobacco cessation, as there is some evidence of efficacy for telephone counseling for this population.

- Maintain up-to-date listings of local cessation programs, as well as a listing of agencies able to help with a range of health and mental health issues, and refer callers to them as appropriate.

- Train staff on resources available to callers in crisis and on when to break confidentiality to ensure safety.

- Provide self-help materials to callers who do not receive counseling, if not to all callers.

Contracting for Quitline Services

Overview

The process of selecting a contractor to provide a quitline service can be lengthy and complex. Careful attention is needed to ensure that state contracting rules and regulations are followed throughout the procurement process. It is prudent to allow at least 6 months from the beginning of the competitive process until a signed contract is in place.

The structure of the request for proposals (RFP) determines the types of information the state will have available for decision making. The statement of work should describe the specific contract deliverables and clearly outline performance expectations and contract deadlines. If these specifications are well defined, it will be much easier to compare proposals.

After the state identifies a successful proposal, the final statement of work and detailed list of deliverables, as well as payment schedules, can be worked out. Contract monitoring begins as soon as the contract is executed and continues throughout the contract period.

This chapter discusses the types of information that should be included in the RFP and briefly describes the proposal review and contract monitoring processes. The case study presented on page 30 details how Washington State procured a vendor for its quitline and how it monitors this contract.

The Request for Proposals

The process for hiring a contractor to operate a statewide quitline is usually guided by the state health department's policies and procedures. Most states require a competitive process, in which the health department issues an RFP and prospective contractors compete with each other to secure the contract. Some states are able to use a noncompetitive selection process to choose a contractor directly, which

> Most states require a competitive process, in which the health department issues an RFP and prospective contractors compete with each other to win the contract.

Contracting for Quitline Services

may save them time. However, these states run the risk of making an uninformed choice, losing power to negotiate terms favorable to the state, or appearing to award contracts for political reasons.

States that elect to use a competitive process must develop an RFP. There are several important considerations for doing so. Most RFPs include a statement of terms and conditions to be imposed on the bidder who wins the contract. These terms and conditions may include standard language from the health department, as well as language restricting the acceptance of tobacco industry funds by the contractor.

The RFP should specify which aspects of the quitline operation are "works for hire" and identify which proprietary products will belong to the contractor. The contracting agency should be aware that the Health Information Portability and Accountability Act (HIPAA) of 1996 may limit its access to data about specific program participants (see Appendix G). Because there is the possibility that the quitline contract may be transferred to another contractor in the future, it is important to determine up front the data management and reporting responsibilities, as well as ownership of all written policies, procedures, and client materials.

In most competitive processes, bidders are asked to prepare at least three specific sections in response to the RFP:

- ◆ A technical proposal that outlines the services to be provided.
- ◆ A management proposal describing the bidder's experience and qualifications to provide quitline services.
- ◆ A budget that may be based on costs, deliverables, or a combination of both.

Questions in the RFP should be framed in an open-ended manner to allow real differences between bidders to emerge.

Questions in the RFP should be framed in an open-ended manner to allow real differences between bidders to emerge. At the same time, the RFP should specify a page limit for each section so that the proposals are concise and easy to compare. Many states request samples of certain deliverables, such as self-help packets, to be mailed to callers and monthly reports to be submitted to the state. Letters of reference may be requested as well.

Once the RFP is written, several steps may be required before its release. The state office of financial management may need to review and approve the document, which can take 10 or more business days. The state may also require that the RFP be announced in a state or local publication.

Contracting for Quitline Services

Many states that have already contracted for quitline services are willing to share the names of organizations that responded to their RFP, and Appendix B lists vendors currently providing such services. Bidders should be allowed at least a month to respond to the RFP. However, if the RFP bundles the operation of the quitline with other activities, such as promotion, bidders will need more time to identify suitable partners.

> Bidders should be allowed at least a month to respond to the RFP—more if they must identify suitable partners.

The Technical Proposal

The technical proposal consists of the statement of work, which spells out the services that the state wants the contractor to provide, and the performance expectations for the contract. The bidder responds by describing how it will provide the requested services. Key items to be addressed in this part of the RFP are outlined in Table 3.1.

Management Proposal

In the management proposal, the bidder describes its experience and capacity to perform the functions outlined in the technical proposal. If requested, letters of reference from other agencies for whom the bidder has provided similar services would be included in this section. Work samples, such as self-help packets and monthly reports, are also requested under this section. Table 3.2 (page 28) lists key items to be addressed.

Budget

The state can ask the bidder to submit a budget that is based on cost-reimbursement, deliverables, or a combination of both. Regulations that govern the use of state or federal funds may specify the type of budget required. It is easier to track expenses in a cost-reimbursement contract, but more difficult to control the total amount spent. In a budget based on deliverables, the bidder sets a price for services that the state pays as the services are delivered. State quitline contracts are frequently a hybrid of the two types of budgets.

It is difficult for vendors to set a unit cost for quitline services because the intensity of service delivery varies greatly between callers, and because the contractor has fixed monthly costs that do not vary as quitline volume varies. It is counterproductive to make bidders guess how much the state is willing to spend on the quitline. Moreover, it might be difficult to compare the resulting proposals. To avoid this situation, the state should disclose budgetary parameters in the RFP. For example, if the state indicates that it plans to spend

> To generate proposals that can be compared with each other, the state should disclose any known budgetary parameters in the RFP.

Contracting for Quitline Services

Table 3.1 Contract Specifications

Services to be provided	Telephone counseling (reactive and/or proactive; average length, average number, timing, and content of sessions; triage system based on readiness to quit and willingness to receive counseling; protocols for special populations) Referral to local programs (including creation and maintenance of resource database) Mailed self-help materials Pharmacotherapy Interactive Web-based programs Information for proxy callers (e.g., wife calling for husband) Technical assistance to health care providers
Hours of operation	Total hours per week Daily and weekly schedule Holidays during which the quitline will be closed Provision for handling calls after hours (e.g., voice mail, answering service)
Target populations	Adults (specify age range) Diverse populations Medicaid and uninsured Youth (specify ages) Pregnant smokers Chewing tobacco users Insured Medicare
Telecommunications standards	Percentage of calls answered live during operating hours Average length of time to live answer Capability to handle multiple simultaneous calls and fluctuations in call volume Voice mail capacity (basic or menu-driven)
Data collection and reporting	Data elements to be collected Backup and recovery of data Security provisions and confidentiality of data Report format, content, and frequency Compliance with HIPAA
Evaluation/quality assurance	Quality improvement plan Staff performance monitoring Quit rate surveys using intent-to-treat analysis and accepted measures Evaluation of reach and effectiveness Satisfaction surveys

Table 3.1 Contract Specifications (continued)

Technology	Strong, scalable communications server
	Automatic call distribution functionality
	Systems that allow real-time monitoring of overall activity as well as individual calls
	Systems to collect, analyze, and report data
	Telephony integration allowing information exchange between voice and data systems
Disaster management	Plans to manage emergencies such as flood, fire, or electrical disruption
Coordination with state health department	Regular meetings with state
	Timely delivery of reports
Quitline marketing (normally the responsibility of the state through its marketing contractor)	Participation in joint planning meetings with marketing contractor
	Advance notice by state for special promotions
	Weekly volume reports to marketing contractor

$500,000 per year on the quitline, bidders can then describe what they would accomplish with that amount of money. This approach also facilitates comparison of the proposals. It is not recommended that states automatically select the lowest bidder, which may represent lower value per dollar spent.

Another issue is how to manage costs to cover inflation over the length of the contract. States often have a fixed amount of funding available each year for quitline services. However, over the life of a multiyear contract, the contracting agency may need to increase its charges based on changes in the local cost of living and other costs. If the state cannot increase the budget in later years, it may be necessary for the contractor to either cut back its level of service or realize cost savings somewhere else in the contract.

It also is important to remember that the contractor does not control monthly call volume. To make the most cost-efficient use of the contract staff, the quitline needs consistent promotion. It is usually the responsibility of the state, not the quitline provider, to market the quitline. Most states assign this responsibility to the media contractor who oversees all anti-tobacco advertising for the state. The state must be sure to budget adequate funds for quitline marketing and to insist on regular communication among all parties. The communication channels between the state, the media agency, and the quitline should be spelled out in the contract.

> To make the most cost-efficient use of the contract staff, the quitline needs consistent promotion.

Contracting for Quitline Services

Table 3.2 Management Proposal Specifications

Experience	Description of experience providing proposed or similar services
Scientific capacity	Familiarity with the science base for quitlines Knowledge of cessation services currently being provided Clinical director on staff Access to scientific advisory board
Management structure, staffing pattern, and qualifications of staff	Organizational charts for parent organization and quitline operator Job descriptions for all positions Resumes of key personnel Sample of monthly staffing schedule
Financial viability	Copy of most recent financial audit
Physical plant	Description of call center workstations and office space Description of network and allocation of servers Description of telephone system, including any software used
System capability and capacity to provide proposed services	Current service delivery levels Additional unused capacity Written policies and procedures for all aspects of operation
Ability to meet contracted time frames	Detailed time line for project planning and implementation, addressing who does what, by when
References	Up to three letters from agencies to which the bidder has provided similar services
Work samples	Samples of products listed as deliverables

Reviewing the Proposals

> A panel of three to seven reviewers should be formed, ideally with expertise in several areas.

Another aspect of the competitive process is preparing to review the proposals once they are received. A panel of three to seven reviewers should be formed. Ideally, each reviewer would have expertise in several areas. Good candidates for the review panel include quitline managers from other states, CDC cessation experts, state staff with expertise in analyzing budgets or experience in implementing similar services (such as drug and alcohol helplines), and agency managers. It is essential to have at least one panel member with a thorough knowledge of the science base for quitlines.

The state must give the review panel clear guidelines on evaluating the proposals. For example, detailed score sheets can be used to ensure a standardized approach (see Appendix E for a sample). Once the proposals have been received and reviewed by the contracts office for completeness, and any nonresponsive proposals eliminated, the remainder should be sent to the reviewers in advance of the scheduled review panel, along with instructions on how to score the proposals using the provided tools. The panel then meets to discuss the proposals and to choose one to recommend for the contract.

Monitoring the Contract

As soon as a contract with the winning bidder is executed, the monitoring process begins. The contract manager is responsible for tracking all deliverables and the contract budget, as well as monitoring the quality of the contractor's performance. Test calls can help the contract manager assess wait time and customer service. Monthly data reports, accompanied by a narrative describing other activities, are essential for contract monitoring. Reports indicating who is calling and at what times calls are being received can be used to modify operations and promotion. In addition, the state should conduct regularly scheduled conference calls and meetings with the contractor. During the first year of operation, such contact may be needed as often as twice a month.

Careful monitoring of service utilization is also critical, because this information is needed to determine any necessary contract modifications. For example, during the first year, utilization of proactive follow-up counseling services and nicotine replacement therapy, if provided, may be substantially higher than what was originally budgeted. Consequently, the state must make decisions about whether to change the budget, the eligibility criteria, or the promotional plan for those services when planning for future years. These decisions have important effects on the future direction and cost of a state's quitline service.

> As soon as a contract with the winning bidder is executed, the monitoring process begins.

Contracting for Quitline Services

Case Study

Contracting Efforts Yield Benefits in Washington State

The process of procuring and working with a contractor can present challenges, but it can also produce favorable results, as it did in Washington State. As this State's story illustrates, it simply takes some time and effort.

In January 2000, 6 months before the start of its funding period, the Washington Department of Health began writing an RFP for a statewide quitline, in consultation with the Centers for Disease Control and Prevention, Office on Smoking and Health (CDC/OSH) and other states that already had quitlines. The RFP was issued in June, with proposals due by mid-July. Several bidders submitted proposals and a review panel was assembled. The panel comprised the Medical Director of Washington State's Uniform Medical Plan, the Quitline Contract Manager from the Oregon Department of Health, a program manager and fiscal officer from the Washington State Department of Health, and a representative of CDC/OSH. The panel recommended the Center for Health Promotion, Inc. (CHP), and this recommendation was quickly approved by the state's Department of Health. CHP was notified of approval at the end of July, and contract negotiations were completed in September. The state negotiated a 3-year contract because it appeared that funding would be stable over that period, and the state wanted to achieve a certain consistency over time in the services provided.

The challenges for Washington State in establishing a quitline have included achieving a contract that meets the needs of both the state and the contractor, negotiating data management issues and production of special reports, and meeting unexpectedly large demand for services, which effectively doubled the contract budget. The quitline was initially planned to provide proactive follow-up to 2,000 clients per year, with fewer than 600 of them receiving nicotine replacement therapy (NRT). However, in its third year of service, the quitline provided proactive follow-up to 3,480 registrants, with 2,822 receiving NRT.

Despite these challenges, the state reports that overall the experience has been positive. Caller satisfaction surveys in the first year indicate that 80% of callers were satisfied with services received and that 70% found the quitline to be helpful in their quitting process. Serious quit attempts were made by 75% of survey respondents, and 12.7% of them were tobacco-free 6 months after they first called.

Note: A link to the RFP and contract developed by Washington State can be found with the online version of this document at http://www.cdc.gov/tobacco.

Contracting for Quitline Services

Recommendations

- ◆ Decide ahead of time which services the contractor will be required to provide, as well as the target populations, evaluation requirements, and available funding. Disclose this information in the RFP.

- ◆ Allow sufficient time for the competitive procurement process—at least 6 months from issuance of the RFP to execution of a contract. Allow bidders at least 1 month to submit their proposals, and more if they must identify partners.

- ◆ Ask bidders to submit (1) a technical proposal describing how they will perform the required functions, (2) a management proposal demonstrating their qualifications, and (3) a detailed budget.

- ◆ Assemble a panel of three to seven proposal reviewers with a range of relevant expertise, including at least one person who has a thorough knowledge of the science base for quitlines. Provide the panel with clear guidelines on how the proposals are to be evaluated.

- ◆ Do not automatically select the lowest bidder. A low-budget proposal may represent lower value per dollar spent.

- ◆ Begin contract management as soon as the contract is signed to ensure optimal performance and to be prepared for any contract modifications that may be needed.

Technological Considerations

Overview

Technologies supporting quitlines are constantly evolving. They have become increasingly powerful and sophisticated and now offer many capabilities that were not widely available when the first quitlines were established. Telephone systems in particular have evolved a set of features specifically for "call centers," the generic term for organizations that conduct a major portion of their business over the telephone, usually from a single location with many agents. Likewise, information systems have evolved many tools for managing the information necessary for the smooth functioning of these call centers.

All states contracting with vendors to provide quitline services should request a complete description of the call-center technology to be used. This chapter examines technologies that are important to quitlines. It also includes a case study that details specific systems and software that the American Cancer Society uses to provide quitline services to several states.

> "Call center" is the generic term for an organization that conducts a major portion of its business over the telephone.

Telephone Systems

Quitlines, like most other call centers, typically utilize a private branch exchange (PBX) telephone system. PBX systems are made by many manufacturers and vary greatly in capacity, but collectively they represent the most robust telephone systems available. All PBX systems have a communications server, which functions as the "brain" of the system. This server can be connected to hundreds or even thousands of telephones. Because such systems lend themselves readily to expansion, quitline providers that are part of larger organizations may simply work within their organization's telephone system instead of buying or leasing a separate one. Quitline providers that do acquire a separate PBX system generally find them easy to scale up as needed.

Technological Considerations

High-speed telecommunication lines enable large amounts of information to be moved efficiently and at low cost.

High-speed telecommunication lines such as T1, DSL (digital subscriber lines), or ISDN (integrated services digital network) enable large amounts of voice or data information to be moved efficiently and at low cost. For the high levels of telephone traffic that quitlines experience, T1 lines provide optimal efficiency. Each T1 line can handle up to 24 simultaneous conversations. Quitline providers can realize savings by using T1 or high-speed lines instead of more expensive, conventional switched-access lines. Also, long-distance rates are cheaper (as low as a few cents per minute) since voice transmissions over T1 lines are less expensive for carriers, and much of the savings is passed through to the subscriber.

Perhaps the most basic call-center function required in a quitline telephone system is the ability to queue incoming calls and route them to staff members according to preestablished priorities. Quitlines that offer service in more than one language need to be able to code each staff member's linguistic abilities in the system so that, for example, calls coming in on a Spanish line are routed only to those who speak Spanish. They may also need to prioritize Spanish calls over English calls if all of their staff members speak English, but only a small number also speak Spanish. This would help address the difference in staffing of the two lines.

A basic call-center function is to queue incoming calls and route them to staff members according to preestablished priorities.

Quitlines may need to define other staff skills in the system, such as the ability to perform intake or to provide counseling. For example, all staff members may be trained in intake, while only a subset is trained to provide counseling. These skills can be programmed into the phone system so that anyone can receive an intake call, but only a counselor can receive a counseling call (e.g., one transferred by an intake worker who has assessed the caller's preference for service). To make the distribution of workload equitable, the system can also be programmed to route calls to the staff member who has gone the longest time without handling a call. These are just a few of the ways in which the "automatic call distributor" (ACD) function of call-center systems enables quitlines to serve large numbers of callers in an organized, efficient manner.

A good telephone system allows supervisors to silently monitor sessions at will.

Quitlines must be able to supervise and monitor the work of their staff, and technology is available to help in this area. A good telephone system allows supervisors to silently monitor sessions at will. This allows the supervisor to ensure that individual staff members provide quality service and to aid them in the event of a crisis, such as when a caller threatens suicide. Training headsets that allow new counselors to shadow a supervisor and hear firsthand how an "expert" counselor handles counseling sessions are available.

Sophisticated software can allow managers to generate a multitude of reports on important aspects of staff members' telephone work, such as the number and length of intake or counseling sessions, percentage of time spent on a call or being available to receive one, percentage of calls answered "live," and so on. Just as important, the software allows real-time monitoring of call traffic, showing at any given moment how many staff members are logged in and available, how many are talking to callers, how many callers are in queue on each toll-free line, how long each has been waiting, and so on.

Some quitlines also use computer telephony integration (CTI), which allows the exchange of information between an organization's voice and data systems. For example, the telephone system can instantly and automatically collect a caller's phone number and route it through the quitline's database to see whether it belongs to a previous caller. If so, the caller's previous records are made available to the current agent, which aids the seamless provision of services. CTI can also make outbound calls more efficient by allowing staff members to speed-dial numbers using their computer mouse. By merging data collected by the telephone system with data collected and entered by staff members, CTI allows quitlines to streamline their processes and improve their performance.

> The merging of data collected by the telephone system with data entered by staff members allows quitlines to streamline processes and improve performance.

Information Systems

Quitline operators need to be able to generate a wide variety of reports, both to ensure high quality in all processes involving interaction with callers and to keep their funding agencies apprised of their activity. Quitline staff typically work within a local area network (LAN) with shared data resources in a centralized database. This allows multiple staff members to interact with the same participants and enter, check, query, and analyze data gathered from them.

Many quitlines develop graphical user interfaces (GUIs) that follow their intake, counseling, and evaluation protocols, essentially serving as computerized survey instruments. The software used to create the front and back ends of quitline databases varies by organization, but almost all applications are proprietary programs created specifically for one quitline contract or another. Reporting capabilities are typically enhanced by inclusion of a standard analysis package such as Statistical Analysis Software (SAS) and a report-generating application such as Crystal Reports.

Technological Considerations

The American Cancer Society's Quitline Demonstrates Effective Use of Technology

In May 2000, the American Cancer Society (ACS) expanded its tobacco-related services by launching a quitline, which is now available in states that contract for this service. The quitline operates out of the ACS National Cancer Information Center (NCIC) in Austin, Texas, and has access to NCIC's state-of-the-art call systems infrastructure and connections.

The ACS quitline has the capacity to meet large spikes in demand resulting from advertising campaigns and events such as the Great American Smokeout. NCIC uses a Siemens telephone and switching system that can handle up to 244 simultaneous incoming and outgoing calls. NIC also uses computer telephony integration software (IBM Call Path and Call Bridge) and workforce management software that help to maximize efficiency. The telephone system supplies ANI (caller location) and DNIS (caller dial-in phone number) data, which allow staff to identify the caller's state-specific quitline program and provide them with geographic and program-specific services. Intake specialists are able to schedule proactive counseling appointments at callers' convenience by using Siebel scheduling software to access counselors' calendars.

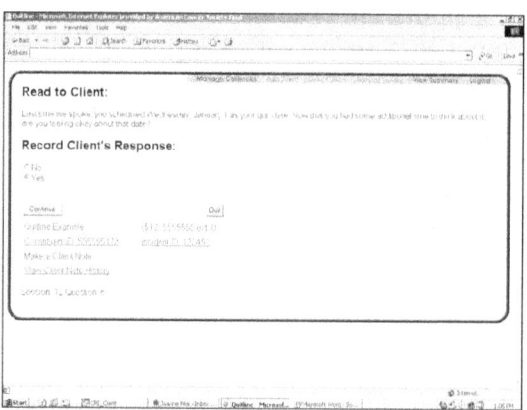

Screen shot of computerized tool used to enter data from intake and counseling calls.

Staff use computerized survey tools to enter data from intake and counseling calls. Every answer to every question is a data point that can be viewed either individually or aggregated with those of other callers for purposes of analysis and reporting. Cold Fusion software is used for data collection and storage, but staff can access the database through Microsoft Access. All data management and cleanup are performed in Access, and then data are exported to SAS for statistical analysis.

Data storage, backup, and recovery procedures are in place to protect all data and programs associated with quitline operation. For example, answers to survey questions are committed to the database after every entry rather than at the end of a session. This enhances the quitline's ability to restore survey data in the event of a system failure.

Technological Considerations

Recommendations

Both the agencies that contract for quitline services and those that provide them should be aware of elements of current call-center technology that can streamline and enhance quitline performance, including

- ◆ Private branch exchange (PBX) telephone systems, which include a strong, scalable communications server capable of serving large numbers of telephones.

- ◆ T1 lines, which are high-speed lines that can handle up to 24 simultaneous calls.

- ◆ Complete automatic call distributor (ACD) functionality to manage the routing of large numbers of calls in an organized, efficient manner.

- ◆ Software that allow supervisors to monitor both individual telephone sessions and overall system activity.

- ◆ Computer telephony integration (CTI), which allows the exchange of information between the voice and data systems.

Staffing a Quitline

Overview

The first step in assessing the appropriate level and types of staffing a contractor should use to operate a quitline is to estimate the intensity, timing, and composition of the call volume that the quitline is likely to receive. This can be accomplished by comparing the planned promotional effort with similar efforts previously conducted within the state or elsewhere. Fortunately, the collective experience among states in promoting and running quitlines provides reference points for estimating the impact of any new promotional effort on the volume of calls.

A primary goal in staffing any organization is to assemble a group of people with the right skills and characteristics for their respective duties. When staffing a quitline, an additional goal is to strike a balance between ensuring that there is enough staff to respond quickly to a sudden wave of incoming calls and ensuring that staff time overall is efficiently engaged in actually helping callers. This chapter addresses ways to achieve these goals.

Staffing for Intake

Staffing Level

A caller's first contact with a quitline typically involves answering some basic questions about smoking status, consumption level, choice of service, and providing other personal and demographic information. Information gathered during the first contact is used to establish a record of the caller in the quitline's database, to which additional data will be added throughout that person's participation in the program. The responsibility for handling and triaging incoming calls falls either to the quitline counselors themselves or, in some cases, to intake specialists. Either way, quitlines must always have sufficient staff available to answer incoming calls during operating hours.

> Reaching a voice mail service rather than a live person can pose a serious barrier for first-time quitline users.

Staffing a Quitline

The number of staff available to answer incoming calls should be based not on the total number of calls received over weeks or months, but on the number needed to respond effectively to the "clusters" of calls that occur immediately after the airing of media spots. Reaching a voice mail system rather than a live person can pose a serious barrier for first-time quitline users, many of whom are experiencing considerable ambivalence about quitting. Although voice mail is often used as a backup when a staff member is not available, many callers will simply hang up rather than leave a message, and it cannot be assumed that they will call a second time. Because the outlay of media dollars required to generate calls can be considerable, it is important from the standpoint of maximizing limited tobacco control resources that the quitline be staffed sufficiently to achieve a high live-answer rate. A quitline that is consistently answering 90% to 95% of calls live during normal hours of operation can be considered to be providing very good coverage.

> A quitline that is consistently answering 90% to 95% of calls live during normal hours of operation can be considered to be providing very good coverage.

Achieving this goal requires coordination with the media campaign so that calls to the quitline are spread across the hours of staff availability to the greatest extent possible. Experienced quitline operators have found that television ads generate calls in clusters and that the quitline may need to have as many as 10 or more staff members available to answer them. (These numbers can vary widely from market to market, depending on the number of people exposed to the ads and other factors discussed in Chapter 9.)

If the quitline fails to achieve at least a 90% live pick-up rate, more intake staff should be made available. The program should also explore ways of spreading out the calls by changing the media plan (for example, by running several less-expensive radio spots instead of one expensive television spot). For quitlines that offer services in more than one language, bilingual staff members are particularly valuable because they provide coverage for two lines.

Staff Skills

> Staff who perform intake must have an excellent telephone manner, good customer service skills, and an ability to triage calls from a wide range of callers.

Staff who perform intake must have an excellent telephone manner, good customer service skills, and an ability to triage calls from a wide range of callers. These include tobacco users who want counseling, those who only want printed materials or referral to a local program, repeat callers who want to speak to a specific counselor, people calling on behalf of a family member, health professionals inquiring about services, students doing school projects, prank callers, and others.

In times of heavy call volume, an intake specialist should be prepared to serve up to 10 or more callers in an hour. This rate is seldom sustained for long, however, because of fluctuations in the call volume. If a quitline employs intake specialists, they can be provided with other duties to be performed when the telephones are not ringing, such as fulfilling requests for mailed materials or calling local programs to make sure referral listings are accurate and up-to-date.

Staffing for Counseling

Most quitlines offer callers who request counseling a first session immediately after intake, whenever possible. This is a straightforward process when the person conducting the intake interview is a counselor. When intake specialists are used, the caller must be transferred to an available counselor. Sometimes, either the caller does not have time for a complete counseling session or a counselor is not available. In these cases, the caller may be scheduled for a later appointment or added to a callback queue for same-day or next-day service.

Staff Skills

Quitlines do not need to be staffed with licensed counselors to have a significant effect on callers' tobacco use. In fact, evidence for the efficacy of proactive quitlines rests mostly on the work of paraprofessional counselors using structured protocols.

Employing staff with basic counseling skills such as empathy, reflective listening, and the ability to guide clients through a structured problem-solving process appears to be key to the success of a quitline. Whether graduate training or extensive clinical experience would impart added benefits is an open question; however, given the desire of most states to fully leverage their limited funds for cessation, it is encouraging that having a successful quitline does not depend on access to the services of comparatively high-paid therapists or other licensed counselors.

There is another reason why it is fortunate that paraprofessionals work well in this position. Quitlines require their counselors to perform the same function repeatedly, and despite the variety in clients' histories and personalities, counseling on a single behavior-modification issue such as smoking cessation can be very repetitive work. For this reason the work may seem too limiting to many professional counselors who have training across a wide range of psychological issues. This can be particularly true in a high-volume, efficiently run quitline.

On the other hand, working as a quitline counselor allows staff who have less formal training or who are concurrently pursuing a graduate

> Evidence for efficacy of proactive quitlines rests mostly on the work of paraprofessional counselors using structured protocols.

degree to gain valuable experience in the field. Counselors who seem to adapt most readily to quitline work are those who have natural counseling skills but not necessarily a strongly developed professional identity as a clinician.

Training

Following up the hiring of candidates who have good natural counseling skills with thorough training is essential. Hiring and training are the most important elements of a quitline's quality assurance program. The initial training program for counselors, prior to allowing them to work with real callers, typically employs a range of formats, including classroom instruction and discussion, live or taped demonstrations of veteran counselors at work, exercises done in groups or pairs, role-playing with fellow trainees or veteran staff, and even an examination. The training programs of some quitlines are comparable in length and scope to college classes, though compressed into the space of a few weeks.

Training programs cover such topics as

- The psychology of tobacco use and the nature of addiction.

- General principles of counseling and theories identified as being helpful in behavior modification, such as cognitive-behavioral counseling and motivational interviewing.

- Other psychological concepts considered useful in understanding tobacco cessation, such as the abstinence violation effect (AVE), a phenomenon in which a single slip triggers a full relapse due to "all-or-nothing" thinking on the part of the quitter.

- Effective counseling techniques, such as reflective listening and paraphrasing.

- Challenging counseling scenarios, including crisis calls, co-morbid conditions, resistant behavior, and callers with psychological issues.

- Ethical and legal guidelines on such issues as mandated reporting and protecting the confidentiality of client information.

- Addressing diversity in clinical work, with respect to culture or ethnicity, education, gender, sexual orientation, religious belief, and other factors.

- Effective case management practices, including use of protocols and tools for setting and keeping appointments.

- Health issues related to tobacco use and cessation.
- Withdrawal.
- NRT and other quitting aids.

Following up the initial training with a regular program of continuing education helps counselors continuously develop their skills and ensures that their knowledge of the field is up to date.

Scheduling

Coordination of counselors' schedules is needed to ensure adequate coverage across the quitline hours of operation. Staffing requirements for different shifts are partially a function of the quitline media campaign, as people tend to call a quitline soon after seeing an ad. It should be noted, however, that many people who call during one shift may actually prefer to receive counseling during another. For example, a smoker who calls the quitline on a break from work may prefer to receive counseling at home in the evening. In such cases, it is helpful if counselors and intake specialists are able to schedule appointments for counselors who work on other shifts. The assigned counselor can then take over to initiate the first session and all subsequent sessions.

Because of the repetitive nature of the work and therefore the "burnout factor," most quitlines hire counselors to work no more than 20 to 30 hours per week. Counselors hired full time may be given supplemental duties so they are not providing counseling 8 hours a day. Expectations of the number of new callers served per counselor vary widely from program to program and depend on numerous factors. These factors include the length and complexity of the counseling protocol used, the number and length of proactive followup sessions to be offered, and whether counselors are also expected to perform intake, take messages for each other, or accomplish other duties. Quitlines typically expect counselors to provide counseling for one to two new clients per hour.

In staffing for both intake and counseling, a quitline must strike a balance between two competing needs. On the one hand, sufficient staff must be available during normal operating hours to serve a wave of new clients calling the quitline in response to an ad. It is not unusual for 10 to 15 people to call within a few seconds of seeing an ad on TV, even though only half may want counseling right away. On the other hand, the quitline cannot afford to have staff sitting idle for too long.

Staffing a Quitline

> Supervisors are responsible for ensuring adequate coverage of calls, timely case management, and high productivity among counselors.

While striking a balance between these two competing needs is challenging for any quitline, it is less so for large quitlines or quitline vendors that serve multiple states. The reason is that at some point in a quitline's growth, the number of counselors who are between counseling sessions at any given moment becomes sufficient to handle a sudden wave of media-generated calls. Assuming that counselors are in session for 40 out of every 60 minutes, at any moment a third of the counselors are free to take a call. If a quitline has six counselors per shift, only two are available to deal with a sudden wave of callers. But if there are 30 counselors per shift, 10 are available to respond should a surge in calls occur. This suggests that as states identify additional resources to grow their quitlines, they will obtain a greater economy of scale and greater efficiency with the additional money.

Staffing for Supervision and Clinical Oversight

Quitlines typically assign 10 to 15 counselors to each supervisor. The supervisors are responsible for ensuring adequate coverage of calls, timely case management, and high productivity among the counselors in their group. They also debrief after difficult calls. A clinical director with expertise in mental health and/or medical issues provides oversight on the appropriateness of the quitline's interventions, both across the board and in particularly challenging situations. An example of the latter would be when a client exhibits evidence of untreated psychopathology. The clinical director also ensures the program's compliance with relevant ethical and legal guidelines that govern the provision of counseling services in that state.

A Contractor's Perspective on Recruitment and Training

Many state agencies, private health plans, and employers that offer quitline services contract with an outside organization to provide them. The Center for Health Promotion, Inc. (CHP), is a major provider of these services, and has well-established procedures for the recruitment and training of new specialists.

CHP requires tobacco cessation specialists to have a bachelor's degree in a health-related field, such as psychology, sociology, social work, community health, or nursing. An associate's degree may be accepted with sufficient professional experience. Applicants must have at least a year of relevant experience, such as crisis line work or one-on-one interviewing; volunteer work is acceptable. They must have been tobacco-free for at least 2 years. Candidates must be able to manage cases using a detailed protocol, and computer skills are required and assessed. Fluency in a foreign language is a plus.

New specialists undergo an intensive 50- to 60-hour training program involving classroom time and practical work on the phone lines. Classroom training covers the science of nicotine addiction, stages of change, intervention techniques, pharmacotherapy, and management of special cases (such as pregnant smokers and callers with other health issues such as asthma, diabetes, cardiopulmonary disease, and depression). Trainees then engage in practical training, which consists of listening to calls handled by experienced staff, participating in role-plays, conducting calls, and debriefing with supervisors and trainers. They also learn the protocols, database applications, and computerized input systems.

Following the training, new specialists are paired with a more experienced specialist who can offer them support and guidance in their new role. For the first couple of months, new specialists are closely monitored, and a standardized tool is used to document and monitor the quality of their calls.

The staffing ratio is one supervisor for every 15 specialists, and at least one supervisor is on duty during each shift. CHP has found that the quality of specialists' work is optimal when they work 20 to 30 hours per week. Specialists are expected to work with two to three callers per hour.

Staffing a Quitline

Recommendations

◆ Refer to other states' experience in promoting and running quitlines to estimate the likely impact of any new promotional effort on a quitline's call volume.

◆ Staff the quitline at a level sufficient to handle the sudden waves or clusters of calls that will follow a TV commercial promoting the quitline, if such ads are used.

◆ Consider including intake specialists in the staffing pattern, but retain the ability to transfer callers to a live counselor if the caller would like counseling right away.

◆ In prospective intake specialists, look for good customer service skills, an excellent telephone manner, and an ability to triage calls from a variety of callers.

◆ Enable intake specialists and counselors to set appointments for other counselors, to serve callers who wish to receive counseling at another time.

◆ In prospective counselors, look for strong, natural counseling skills rather than advanced degrees or licensure.

◆ Provide intensive on-the-job training for counselors that utilizes a range of instructional modalities and covers a broad range of relevant topics.

◆ To avoid counselor burnout, hire counselors at 20 to 30 hours per week or provide them with supplemental duties so that they do not have to counsel 8 hours a day.

◆ A clinical director with mental health and/or medical expertise should provide clinical oversight and ensure compliance with ethical and legal guidelines.

Quality Assurance in Quitline Counseling

Overview

Quality assurance is important in all public health organizations, but especially in those offering behavioral interventions based on clinical research findings. Clinical trials are usually conducted in the context of strict quality control. When the findings from these trials are applied in a real-world setting, quality control may be significantly less stringent. With less vigilance in this area, the intervention's effectiveness may suffer. Although the evidence demonstrating the efficacy of quitlines is strong, effectiveness in all quitlines is not guaranteed. For this reason, and given the increasing public investment in quitlines, it is vital that states and their quitline operators closely monitor quality.

> It is vital that states and their operators closely monitor quality.

This chapter provides information on ensuring the quality of the counseling provided by quitline staff and recommendations for developing a quality improvement plan. Also included in this chapter is a case study that details the quality assurance practices of the Mayo Clinic Tobacco Quitline.

Quality Assurance in Daily Operations

As discussed in Chapter 5, recruiting qualified counselors and providing thorough training are two of the most important elements of a good quality assurance program for quitlines. Regular quality monitoring of the services provided by these counselors is equally important and is a key function of the quitline's internal management structure. Several tools are available for this purpose.

Supervision

Comprehensive supervision is a key component of quality assurance. Attention to both competency and productivity is necessary to

> Attention to both competency and productivity is necessary to maintain a consistently high level of performance.

Quality Assurance in Quitline Counseling

maintain a consistently high level of performance. To ensure effectiveness, supervisors should fulfill the following responsibilities:

- Oversee the content and delivery of counseling sessions.
- Monitor calls.
- Conduct debriefing sessions.
- Work with counselors to improve their clinical strengths in the areas of behavior modification and addictions treatment.
- Oversee case management.

In addition, to ensure timeliness and efficiency, a supervisor should meet regularly with each counselor in his or her unit to review performance statistics. These statistics may include the following:

- Number and percentage of callers who received counseling.
- Number and timing of follow-up sessions per client.
- Average length of sessions.
- Number of attempts to reach clients for outgoing calls.
- Percentage of time logged into the telephone system and available for incoming calls.
- Percentage of calls answered live and within a set time limit (e.g., 20 seconds).
- Other performance measures tied to the quitline's protocols.

> Protocols serve as training tools and mechanisms for quality assurance.

Use of Protocols

Many quitlines establish specific protocols for working with different subgroups of callers. Protocols also vary with respect to how fully scripted they are and how closely counselors are required to follow them. They are powerful mechanisms for quality assurance that serve as training tools for new counselors, define the minimum acceptable content for each session, and guide the flow of the discussion.

Protocols also serve as a consistent reminder to the counselor of the clinical issues considered to have the most bearing on quitting success. They help the counselor to be comprehensive in his or her attention to the relevant issues, but also brief and focused. Several quitlines use versions of protocols that were shown to be effective in trials of telephone counseling for smoking cessation. Some quitlines are testing new protocols for special populations.

Quality Assurance in Quitline Counseling

Peer Feedback

Another avenue for quality assurance is to encourage counselors to give and receive peer feedback. Most quitline counselors work in open office environments where they continually overhear each other speaking with clients. That means they are in a good position to help ensure the accuracy of information provided to callers, as well as adherence to protocols. Counselors can provide each other with constructive feedback on an informal basis or discuss issues more formally during staff meetings. Some quitlines hold regular group supervision meetings for more formalized exchange of peer feedback. In these meetings, challenging clinical issues also can be raised and case studies may be examined for lessons learned.

Evaluation

Almost all quitlines are continually evaluated to some extent. At a minimum, this usually involves telephone follow-up surveys with randomly selected callers after they have participated in the program. Interviewers collect objective behavioral data such as smoking status, as well as more subjective satisfaction data.

Such surveys may contain specific questions about the callers' experience with their counselors, and the answers to these questions can be shared anonymously with the counselors who worked with them. Callers' assessments of the quality of service they received can help counselors improve their performance and acknowledge them for a job well done. Chapter 7 provides more information on evaluation.

Quality Improvement

Although the contract manager is unlikely to be involved in the daily particulars of quality assurance within the contractor's organization (for example, giving feedback to individual counselors), he or she must ensure that the contractor is following a comprehensive quality improvement plan.

The quality improvement plan should describe the procedures, standards, and measures to be used to ensure quality. It should also discuss how the organization's performance in the various areas of quality assurance is to be reported, how the reported data should be interpreted, and how that information will be used not only to maintain the quality of services but to improve them as well. States may want to consider how to build incentives into their quitline contracts for achievement of agreed-upon benchmarks or measurable improvements over time.

Quality Assurance in Quitline Counseling

Mayo Clinic Tobacco Quitline Is Guided by Strict Quality Assurance Practices

Attention to program protocols is key to the quality assurance practices of the Mayo Clinic Tobacco Quitline.[1] Counselors follow general smoking cessation protocols and protocols for special populations, though they can also consult with Mayo Clinic physicians and other counselors concerning issues not directly addressed by the protocols. The protocols are adjusted as research-based data become available, and additional training is provided as needed.

Collection and analysis of call data also are critical to ensuring quality. The quitline's database permits call volume and utilization analysis by the hour, day, week, and month. Collective performance standards to ensure that the organization is providing timely service include the following:

- A call abandonment rate of no more than 5%.
- 95% of calls answered within 30 seconds.
- 100% of messages returned within 1 business day.
- 100% of quit kits mailed within 48 hours.
- 50% requesting immediate counseling receive it.

The work of individual counselors is periodically evaluated for clinical quality. A review tool is used to assess their performance with an individual client, and addresses whether they

- Conducted a complete assessment of the caller.
- Provided complete and accurate information on session content, confidentiality, treatment options (including nicotine replacement therapies and use of support systems), and relapse.
- Confirmed the follow-up appointment.
- Presented all information in a professional and nonjudgmental manner and used open-ended questions and language appropriate to the caller's level of understanding.

The quitline also obtains satisfaction and outcome data through evaluation follow-up calls with a sample of program participants. To ensure that these data are not compromised by the counselor-client relationship, these calls are conducted by intake assistants. The quitline's management staff uses the data to identify areas for improvement and report on progress toward these goals. The quitline manager, a leadership team, and a continuous improvement committee review the data before finalization of the report. Trends are noted, and any complex or indeterminate data are identified and reviewed with Mayo Clinic Nicotine Dependence Center physicians and the quitline coordinator.

---

1 Mayo Clinic Tobacco Quitline is a telephone-based tobacco intervention product of MMSI, a Mayo health company and Mayo Foundation subsidiary.

Recommendations

- Ensure that counselors receive comprehensive supervision that addresses both clinical issues (e.g., knowledge of effective behavior modification techniques) and administrative issues (e.g., efficiency and productivity in case management).

- Use evidence-based counseling protocols.

- Provide formal and informal opportunities for counselors to receive constructive feedback from their peers.

- Review with counselors the outcome and satisfaction data gathered by the evaluation staff.

- Develop and follow a quality improvement plan describing quality assurance procedures, standards, and measures for tracking the program's performance; how performance will be reported and interpreted; and how quality will be improved over time.

Evaluating a Quitline

Overview

The evaluation of a quitline has three main functions: (1) it provides information that can help improve services; (2) it creates an accountability mechanism for the contractor; and (3) it provides information to the contracting agency on the quantity, quality, and value of services provided. Evaluation can include a needs assessment, permitting the program to adjust its activities to the needs of the field. It can include process evaluation, providing an account of program activities to let the funding agency or others outside the project understand what is being done. Evaluation can also include an analysis of effectiveness, providing outcome data that help justify the existence of the quitline and inform the field about the effectiveness of certain interventions.

Adding evaluation to a quitline's required activities naturally increases the workload, but a significant part of the evaluation can be accomplished while the quitline is providing services, if the program keeps careful records along the way. For example, most quitlines send self-help materials to callers. To receive these materials, callers must provide their mailing addresses, which include ZIP codes. ZIP codes can be a good proxy measure for household income, since socioeconomic profiles are available for each ZIP code. Thus, within the task of recording data to provide good service lies an opportunity to measure how well the program is doing with respect to reaching a socioeconomically diverse population.

The content and intensity of evaluation activities are dictated by the goals of the quitline, which may differ from one state to another. The following list of general content questions can help shape the evaluation activities of most quitlines. Appendix F contains a more detailed matrix that can be used when designing an evaluation plan.

◆ What is the purpose of the quitline?

◆ What populations is the quitline intended to serve?

Evaluating a Quitline

- What types and quantities of service does the quitline provide?
- What are the effects of quitline services?
- How satisfied are quitline callers with the services provided?
- How much does the quitline contribute to the larger program of tobacco control?

In addition to examining these content questions, this chapter discusses logistical issues that must be addressed, such as the timing of evaluations and who will conduct them.

Elements Shaping the Evaluation Plan

Purpose of the Quitline

The purpose of a quitline is usually established by the funding agency when it issues its request for proposals (RFP). Quitlines may be created to augment health provider advice, to target specific groups such as pregnant smokers, to act as frontline sources of quick stop-smoking advice and to triage callers back to their health plans or to local programs, or to provide comprehensive cessation services to anyone who requests them. Whatever the focus, variables selected for evaluating a quitline's services should be linked to the purpose of the quitline.

> Variables selected for evaluating a quitline's services should be linked to the purpose of the quitline.

Most existing statewide quitlines are established to provide a variety of services for a diverse group of callers, ranging from mailed self-help information to proactive counseling. Underlying this general purpose, there are usually subobjectives that can be stated in measurable terms, preferably with predetermined benchmarks to compare performance over time (for example, the percentage of tobacco users of ethnic minority backgrounds served by the quitline). These subobjectives should be established at an early stage in the project.

Often, statewide quitlines are used in conjunction with anti-smoking media campaigns, with the assumption that the two activities will support each other. In this case, the evaluation must consider how and to what extent the quitline supports the goals of the media campaign (for example, by helping to address geographic disparities in tobacco use and access to effective treatment).

Evaluation data also may indicate a need to modify the quitline's objectives. For example, a quitline that is specifically designed to serve teenage smokers and that targets this age group through its promotional efforts may find that it is receiving many more calls from adults than from teens. The contracting agency would need this information to make an informed decision about whether to modify the original goals of the project. (See Appendix F: *Proposed Minimal Data Set for Evaluation* for guidance.)

Target Populations

The most basic evaluation of a quitline simply describes its users. This includes demographic information such as age, gender, and ethnicity. A basic evaluation may also assess other relevant information such as level of tobacco use, quitting history, intention to quit, exposure to secondhand smoke, and restrictions on smoking at home. Because information about these variables is useful for clinical intervention as well as for evaluation purposes, it should be collected when tobacco users first call the quitline, as part of the intake process.

It is useful to compare the tobacco users who call the quitline with those in the state's general population. This gives a sense of how well the quitline and its promotional campaign are doing in reaching the target populations. For example, if 20% of a state's tobacco users are Latino, then a quitline receiving 20% or more of its calls from members of the Latino community is doing well in this regard. However, if the percentage of calls from a target population is lower than its proportion among the state's tobacco users, then a more targeted promotional strategy may be needed. Information such as this is crucial for making informed decisions about how best to reach out to the state's priority populations. With that in mind, it also is beneficial to ask callers, at their first call, how they heard about the quitline.

For a new quitline, a comparison of its data with data from other quitlines of a similar nature can be informative. For example, if a quitline with a specific goal of reaching geriatric smokers determines that a much smaller percentage of this population than anticipated has called the quitline, it would be useful to compare its data with data from other quitlines that also target older smokers. Using data gathered from a number of states should help to develop a realistic estimate of the percentage of older smokers who will use a quitline or to identify specific promotional strategies that have been successful in reaching this population.

Evaluating a Quitline

Types and Quantities of Services Provided

After determining basic information about callers, the next step is to conduct a process evaluation of services provided, the intensity of each service, and the percentage of callers receiving each service. It is important to start the process evaluation by defining terms. For example, what constitutes a call to the quitline? Does a hang-up count as a call? Should each access to a taped message be counted as a separate caller? What counts as counseling? Should callers who ask specific questions about cessation but do not identify themselves be counted as having received counseling? Is there a minimum length of time before a conversation can be counted as counseling? How many sessions constitute a multiple counseling protocol? All such terms need to be carefully defined.

Established quitlines generally offer a range of services and let the callers decide what services they prefer. Monitoring the use of various quitline services provides important information for making decisions concerning service delivery. For example, counseling is the most labor-intensive activity of all quitline services, so the percentage of callers opting for this service can significantly affect the cost of the quitline operation. Furthermore, the proportion of smokers opting for and receiving a particular service can vary widely from one quitline to another. The New York and Wisconsin quitlines offer callers the options of speaking with a trained counselor, leaving their name and address to receive a packet of self-help materials in the mail, or listening to taped messages. In New York, roughly a third of callers opt for each of these three services. In Wisconsin, on the other hand, more than 75% of callers opt for counseling in addition to receiving the mailed packet (McAfee 2002).

In addition to documenting service utilization, an evaluation also can examine factors that influence a caller's choice of service. Few first-time callers to a quitline, especially those responding to a media campaign, have a clear idea of what services are provided or what it means to receive counseling by telephone. As a result, their service preference may be affected by the way the quitline presents its menu of services. Other factors, such as the working hours of counselors and the intensity of counseling, may also influence callers' choice of services.

An improved understanding of the factors affecting callers' choice of services (based on the evaluation results) can help the contracting agency and its provider to manage the quitline's workload (for example, by controlling the total number of callers going into counseling or by improving its ability to recruit smokers into more intensive treatment). Effective workload management aids in maintaining high service quality and efficient utilization of resources, especially during unexpected fluctuations in call volume.

Effects of Service

One of the most important steps in evaluating quitlines is to determine how many callers actually quit using tobacco and to what extent, if any, this can be attributed to the quitline's services. Outcome data help to justify the program's efforts and to inform the field about whether certain interventions are actually working.

Again, defining terms is important, especially defining what counts as a "quit." Multiple measures have been used in the scientific literature; they range from having quit for at least 1 day (at a certain point of follow-up) to having quit for at least 12 months (Velicer et al. 1992, Hughes et al. 2003). The Society for Research on Nicotine and Tobacco recently published a consensus paper on measuring quitting success in intervention trials (Hughes et al. 2003) that recommends continuous nonsmoking at 6 or 12 months as the main outcome measure for clinical interventions, with other periods of abstinence as secondary measures (e.g., being abstinent for 7 or 30 days at 6- or 12-month follow-up).

Absolute quit rates will differ significantly, depending on which measure is used to define a successful quit. Quitlines using stricter definitions, such as 12-month continuous abstinence, may appear to have lower absolute quit rates than those with less stringent definitions, such as 7-day point prevalence (the percentage of participants who have been abstinent for 7 days at follow-up). Published studies from across the field are often inconsistent with each other in their definitions of quitting, but it is important that each state be consistent at least within its own documents. Once the measure of a successful quit is chosen, the simplest approach is to calculate the percentage of quitline callers who have quit smoking by a particular point in time (for example, 6 months after their initial call). This provides a general idea of how successful callers are in quitting.

The limitation of using such a simple approach for outcomes evaluation is that it cannot in itself determine what proportion of the quitting is attributable to the quitline's assistance and what proportion would have occurred without it. To identify the proportion of the quit rate that is attributable to the quitline's services would require a randomized controlled study, but denying services to members of a control group for evaluation purposes is, of course, undesirable in a service setting.

> Outcome data help to justify the program's efforts and to inform the field about whether certain interventions are actually working.

> Defining terms is important, especially what counts as a "quit."

Evaluating a Quitline

In certain service settings, a method has been developed to separate the quitline's counseling effects from the overall quit rates without denying services to a group of callers (Zhu et al. 2002). However, most quitlines can obtain only a simple quit rate without a comparison control group. In these cases, there are specific issues that the evaluation report should address to clarify readers' understanding of the reported quit rates (see box below).

Reporting Quit Rates

Quit rates can vary dramatically depending on how they are calculated. When there is no randomized control group for comparison, an evaluation report must clearly address certain issues so that the results can be interpreted correctly. Specifically, the report should

- ◆ Provide a complete account of how callers contacting the quitline were selected for the evaluation sample, since the quit rate can change dramatically depending on who was excluded.
- ◆ Describe any baseline caller characteristics in the evaluation sample that may predict quitting success or failure, such as the number of cigarettes smoked and intention to quit.
- ◆ Provide a long-term continuous abstinence rate for a random sample of all participants who agreed to receive counseling, calculated by dividing the number of participants who report that they have not used tobacco for a stated length of time (e.g., 6 or 12 months) by the number of participants who were reached for follow-up.
- ◆ Specify the contact rate for the evaluation sample, because loss to follow-up can also affect the quit rate.
- ◆ Provide an additional analysis assuming that those lost to follow-up were still using tobacco (i.e., the number of participants who report that they have not used tobacco for a stated length of time divided by the number of participants who were selected for the evaluation sample) regardless of whether they were successfully followed up.

Failure to address these issues when there is no control group will greatly hamper readers' ability to interpret reported quit rates in a meaningful way.

Caller Satisfaction

Another important outcome is caller satisfaction. Data on how satisfied callers were with the service they received can become part of the public record and often weigh heavily in policy and funding decisions. In addition, regular monitoring of user satisfaction yields information that can be used to improve services, thus increasing the satisfaction of future users.

A simple method for obtaining satisfaction data is to directly survey a random sample of smokers receiving each of the quitline services (self-help materials, taped messages, personal counseling, and so on). The surveys can include open-ended questions that are designed to elicit more detailed opinions, such as: "What was your experience when you first called the quitline?" "Were the materials useful?" "Was your counselor a good listener?" "Was he or she knowledgeable about how to quit smoking?" "Is there anything else the quitline should be doing?"

Another way of monitoring caller satisfaction is to study callers' complaints about the quitline. While not all complaints are legitimate (for example, a smoker may complain that his counselor did not call him, when in fact the counselor did call, but the smoker failed to keep the appointment), some callers will have a less than satisfactory experience. Because not all dissatisfied callers lodge complaints, paying careful attention to every complaint that is received can help prevent the spread of dissatisfaction stemming from hidden problems in the program.

The Quitline's Contribution to the Tobacco Control Program

So far, the discussion of evaluation has focused on the quitline's role in providing clinical services. However, a statewide quitline is usually a key part of a larger tobacco control program, so it is important to assess the quitline's contribution to the overall effort to reduce tobacco use in the general population. It is very difficult to quantify precisely the contribution of one particular element of a larger tobacco control program because these programs intentionally mix elements to produce synergy (Fishbein et al. 2000). However, there are several considerations that will help in evaluating the population impact of a quitline.

The first of these concerns the direct impact of the quitline. The total direct effect of a quitline on the tobacco-using population is the product of the number of callers and the efficacy of the service. If a quitline maintained its effectiveness regardless of the number of calls, then the effect of the quitline on the population would be in direct proportion to the percentage of smokers calling.

Most state quitlines currently reach 1% to 5% of their states' total tobacco-using population in any given year. The fact that their reach is not wider than this is generally due to funding constraints that require quitlines to restrict services, promotion, or both. Increasing the funding would increase the percentage of smokers reached, which would in turn increase the total direct impact of the quitline. But without an increase in funding, any substantial increase in the call volume requires efforts to balance the effectiveness of the service with the capacity of the quitline to handle the increased volume. To increase the capacity of the quitline to handle more calls without incurring extra cost, the intensity of treatment for each smoker may need to be reduced, which may lead to lower effectiveness per caller. Even so, a lower-efficacy intervention protocol handling a greater number of callers can be more cost-effective than a higher-efficacy protocol handling fewer callers. Careful evaluation is needed to help locate the balancing point that would allow the quitline to achieve the maximum direct impact with a given amount of funding.

A second issue to consider when assessing the population impact of a quitline is that a quitline's actual reach may be greater than the number of tobacco users who call. Many more smokers will hear the media promotion than will call the quitline. In one controlled study, only about a third of all smokers who knew about the quitline actually called (Ossip-Klein et al. 1991). However, the overall quit attempt rate among the group that knew about the quitline was greater than among the group that did not know about the service, suggesting that awareness of the quitline had some impact even on the smokers who did not call. More studies testing such indirect quitline effects are needed.

A third issue to consider is the potential synergy between state quitlines and other elements of comprehensive programs. The hope in any comprehensive approach is that the combined effect will be greater than the sum of the effects of individual program components. One version of the synergy hypothesis is that the availability of a quitline increases the effect of an anti-tobacco media campaign on the prevalence of tobacco use. That is, if the monies spent on the quitline were instead used to expand the media campaign, the total effect on prevalence would be smaller. Although no study has tested this hypothesis, it is noteworthy that the states with the sharpest reductions in tobacco consumption (California, Massachusetts, Arizona, and Oregon) have all invested in comprehensive tobacco control programs, including both quitlines and aggressive media campaigns (Farrelly 2003).

Logistical Issues

Timing

The timing of an evaluation activity should be determined by its purpose and the kinds of information that are to be collected. As mentioned earlier, evaluation can start as early as the first contact with callers, when they provide information about themselves in order to receive services. In addition to basic demographic information, other examples of data to collect at baseline include daily (or weekly) tobacco consumption and how soon after waking one smokes, both of which are dependence measures. It is usually a good idea to obtain as much information as possible at initial contact, as long as it does not interfere with service delivery. This is particularly important for variables that change over time (for example, callers' confidence in their ability to quit smoking), so that baseline information is available for later comparison.

> Evaluation can start as early as the first contact with callers, when they provide information about themselves in order to receive services.

It is probably best to conduct a simple assessment of user satisfaction soon after service is delivered. But when conducting a formal evaluation of quit rates, it is important to ensure that participants do not confuse evaluation calls with counseling calls. Toward this end, it is helpful to plan for a "break" of at least a month between the last call in the counseling protocol and the first call in the evaluation protocol. To obtain accurate information on relapses, repeated quit attempts, changes in social environment, and so on, repeated evaluation calls may be needed.

Whereas data gathered by an impartial evaluation team after service is complete are crucial to the quitline evaluation effort, many questions can be answered by simply describing the quitline population and its utilization of services, as described earlier. Much data can be collected while service is being delivered. For this reason, the importance of careful data management cannot be overstated. States should define what they want to know from the evaluation early on, and should work with their independent evaluator (if they have one) and the quitline management staff to ensure that the database is set up early in the process and that it includes all of the variables that will be needed for evaluation, facilitating future analysis.

> The importance of careful data management cannot be overstated.

Although evaluation is best started early and continued throughout the program, it is neither cost-efficient nor necessary to evaluate every participant. Most state quitlines serve thousands of callers. In these cases, it is necessary to evaluate only a random sample of participants. Only if a quitline were serving a very small number of callers would evaluation of all participants be indicated.

Evaluating a Quitline

> Valuable evaluation work can be done in-house, but it is important that the evaluation staff be distinct from the intervention staff.

Evaluation Staff Selection

There is a general belief that only people outside the project can be impartial evaluators. Some state funding agencies prefer to have evaluations conducted or at least overseen by people who are not part of the quitline staff. However, valuable evaluation work can also be done in-house. Intervention researchers (and medical researchers) routinely evaluate the effects of treatments they have designed, and there are ethics guidelines to govern this scientific conduct. However, if a quitline contractor is evaluating its own intervention, it is important that the evaluation staff at least be distinct from the intervention staff. The reason is that even if the intervention staff can be objective during evaluations, the program participants may be biased to give socially desirable answers if the person evaluating their quitting success is also the person who delivered the service.

A benefit of conducting follow-up evaluation calls in-house, especially those aimed at improving quitline services, is that the evaluation staff can work closely with the intervention staff to identify important issues and to design questionnaires that will address those issues immediately. Evaluation is not just a passive process of accounting for what has happened but also an active research process that helps a quitline to be continuously innovative, identifying new strategies to help smokers and expanding its service to new areas.

Recommendations

◆ Make evaluation an integral component of quitline operations, as it helps both to keep the program accountable and to improve service.

◆ Build evaluation into the program from the beginning, by articulating the goals and subgoals of the quitline, identifying benchmarks, and deciding on the essential data to be gathered.

◆ Require quitline staff to keep careful records and, in so doing, to accomplish a significant portion of the evaluation.

◆ In evaluating a quitline, examine how well it is reaching its target populations, types and quantities of services provided, effects of the service, caller satisfaction, and its contribution to the broader tobacco control program.

Evaluating a Quitline

- When reporting results, provide a detailed description of the process of choosing the sample of participants to be evaluated, the contact rate for follow-up, the long-term continuous abstinence rate for those who were reached for follow-up, and an additional analysis assuming that all those lost to follow-up were still using tobacco.

- Specify whether those who could not be followed up were excluded from the analysis.

- Be consistent when using definitions and measures for quitting behavior.

Costs Associated with Operating a Quitline

Overview

As noted earlier, most quitlines operate not as stand-alone clinical services, but as part of a comprehensive tobacco control program. Thus, estimating costs for a quitline depends partly on the role that it is expected to play in the larger program. For example, is it designed to augment the mass media campaign's cessation messages by providing a low-cost service to a large number of callers? Or is it intended to provide more intensive, comprehensive counseling to a smaller number of callers? Is it meant to provide comprehensive treatment to any smoker desiring assistance, or a safety net for those unable to access the health care system? The answers to these types of questions have great bearing on cost calculations because they define the service structure of the quitline, which in turn affects costs.

> Estimating costs for a quitline depends partly on the role that it is expected to play in the larger tobacco control program.

This chapter examines the costs of quitlines from two perspectives. The first focuses on the internal structure of a quitline budget, that is, the percentage of funds dedicated to various key activities within the organization. The second focuses on the cost of a quitline in relation to the costs of other activities within the tobacco control program.

Estimating Annual Costs by Key Activities

A quitline generally engages in three key activities:

◆ Intake (handling incoming calls from new program participants and mailing self-help materials).

◆ Counseling.

◆ Evaluation.

In addition, there are important support activities. One is coordination with promotional efforts. (Since mass media promotion is generally handled by a separate agency, a separate media budget must be developed.) Other activities include providing administrative

> Most quitlines can expect to spend between 65% and 80% of their operational budgets on intake and counseling.

Telephone Quitlines: *A Resource for Development, Implementation, and Evaluation*   65

Costs Associated With Operating a Quitline

support for the project as a whole; providing technical support for telephone, database, and computing facilities; managing clearinghouse services; and conducting training.

Most states can expect to spend between 65% and 80% of their operational budgets on intake and counseling. If the primary objective of a new quitline is to provide comprehensive, proactive counseling (which is the model followed by most U.S. quitlines), intake can be expected to require about 10% to 15% of the budget, counseling about 55% to 65%, and evaluation about 10%. The remaining funds will go toward staff training, development of materials, and in-house promotional activities (assuming that the bulk of media promotion is handled by a separate organization, as is usually the case). The costs of providing administrative and technical support are subsumed within each category.

If, on the other hand, the primary objective of a quitline is to provide brief, reactive counseling to a larger number of callers (in the manner of a hotline), the line between intake and counseling blurs. However, the total proportion of the budget dedicated to both activities will probably remain between 65% and 80%, which differs little from a quitline operating under a proactive counseling model.

> Evaluation is critical for the overall health of the program, and funding for this activity should be considered a key component of a responsible quitline budget.

Many states have allocated about 10% of their quitline budgets to evaluation. As discussed in Chapter 7, evaluation is critical for the overall health of the program, and funding for this activity should be considered a key component of a responsible quitline budget. In conceptualizing the scope of evaluation, it is helpful to try to foresee what information would be needed if one had to justify the quitline's continued existence.

A question that frequently arises with respect to the calculation of quitline costs is how much it costs to counsel a single tobacco user (McAlister et al. 2004). The answer depends on several factors, including the cost of living in the area where the quitline is located, the educational background of the staff providing the service, whether medications are provided, and operational efficiency. But the key variable is the relative comprehensiveness of the counseling provided.

> There is no generally applicable calculation of cost per person counseled because the counseling protocols of existing quitlines vary widely in length and intensity.

There is no generally applicable calculation of cost per person counseled because the counseling protocols of existing quitlines vary widely in length and intensity. For proactive counseling protocols, which usually aim to provide four to six calls per person, the total cost per person counseled ranges from $175 to $230, although these calculations sometimes include the cost of evaluating a sample of callers. For reactive counseling protocols, a per-person figure is not available; however, it obviously costs less to provide brief, reactive counseling sessions than to provide more intensive, proactive sessions.

Another important question for a state quitline is what amount represents a minimum acceptable level of funding. Reasonable funding for a state quitline ensures that the operation is staffed at a level sufficient to allow it to serve as a meaningful component of the state's comprehensive tobacco control program. A quitline has many advantages that make it particularly well suited to play an important role in a state's comprehensive tobacco control program. For example, it provides a very convenient cessation service. However, if a statewide quitline is insufficiently promoted or insufficiently staffed, its fitness for that role is diminished.

In 2001, the median annual budget for U.S. quitlines was $600,000 (Zhu 2002a), not including the cost of promotion. The amount of funding required in a given state depends in large part on the size of the state's tobacco-using population. A crude method of calculating a minimum funding level is to assume that 2% of the state's adult tobacco users will call the quitline each year, and then to multiply that number by $130. (The figure $130, given in 2004 dollars, comes from multiplying the lowest cost per caller estimate [$175] by about 75%, assuming that 25% of callers will not use counseling.) When this method of calculation is used to compare states that currently have quitlines, it shows that states with larger populations are generally spending less money on their quitlines (per tobacco user in the state) than states with smaller populations.

> In 2001, the median annual budget for U.S. quitlines was $600,000, not including the cost of promotion.

Assessing the Cost of a Quitline in Relation to Other Tobacco Control Costs

A new statewide quitline is usually highly dependent on mass media promotion to inform smokers of its existence (see Chapter 9). Therefore, the advertising budget is closely linked to the budget for operations. Because media spots for the quitline are often purchased with other anti-smoking media spots, it can be difficult to separate the exact amount spent to promote the quitline. Still, a rough estimate can help to set an operating budget for the quitline. For a new quitline, a rule of thumb is to allocate one dollar for quitline operations for every dollar spent on promotion.

> For a new quitline, a rule of thumb is to allocate one dollar for quitline operations for every dollar spent on promotion.

Costs Associated With Operating a Quitline

When considering the costs of quitline operation in relation to those of other anti-smoking activities, the following observations regarding promotion are relevant. First, given the same promotional efforts, smokers are more likely to use a quitline than to use face-to-face clinical services. In a recent survey, smokers were several times more likely to say they would prefer using a quitline to attending a group clinic when the availability of both services was simultaneously made known to them and both were free of charge (McAfee 2002). This suggests that it is significantly less costly to recruit the same number of tobacco users into quitline counseling than to recruit them into traditional cessation clinics.

Second, there may be periods when quitline promotion must be curtailed to keep the number of callers from overwhelming the staff. The "problem" of having too many tobacco users calling for service contrasts with the experience of many traditional cessation group programs, which often have more trained facilitators than needed because of the low number of tobacco users attending.

These observations suggest that, in most cases, there is the potential to increase the size of quitline operations, since additional promotion of quitlines is likely to result in large numbers of smokers using the service. Of course, operational expansion of the quitline requires increased funding. The amount allocated for a quitline often represents a large portion of a state's funding for cessation. However, the amount allocated for cessation usually represents only a small portion of a state's total funding for tobacco control. In other words, states provide little money for cessation, but much of what they do provide for this purpose is entrusted to quitlines.

If a state needs to give its media campaign wider exposure or needs to reach more tobacco users through the quitline, but increased funding for quitline expansion is not feasible, it has the option of making quitline counseling protocols less intensive, so that counseling can be provided to more smokers. The lower-intensity counseling in such a setting probably produces less effect per caller than higher-intensity counseling. However, the total impact on the smoking population may be significant if the lower-intensity counseling protocol allows the program to handle more calls. The total direct effect of a quitline is the product of the number of people who use it and the average effect per person, so the impact of a quitline could theoretically be maintained even with lower-intensity counseling.

> The total direct effect of a quitline is the number of people who use it and the average effect per person.

Costs Associated With Operating a Quitline

Over the long term, however, there will be more quitline callers who relapse in their quit attempts when a lower-intensity intervention is used, which may damage the quitline's credibility as an effective cessation strategy. Therefore if additional funding becomes available, a more desirable option for increasing the impact of the quitline might be to maintain the counseling protocol at a high level of intensity and to increase the program's capacity to serve callers. This approach allays justifiable concerns that abbreviating the protocols may compromise program effectiveness.

Most existing quitlines employ a mixture of reactive and proactive counseling and other services of varying costs in an attempt to use funding as efficiently as possible. Efficient use of funding is an evolving issue even for states with extensive experience with quitlines. It would be a mistake to compare programs on the basis of simple numbers such as cost per call without first carefully examining the whole service protocol and the rationale for each component. Moreover, the smoking population and the makeup of quitline callers change over time, so even states with well-established quitlines should periodically assess their services and associated cost structures in the context of the larger tobacco control agenda.

> States should periodically assess quitline services and costs in the context of the larger tobacco control agenda.

Recommendations

◆ Use the following guidelines to establish a minimum budget for a state quitline:

  - For a new quitline, the operating budget should equal the amount being allocated for the promotion component of the quitline.

  - A crude method of calculating a minimum funding level for operations is to assume that 2% of the state's adult smokers will call the quitline each year, and then to multiply that number by $130.

  - Currently, the median annual budget for state quitlines is about $600,000.

  - The cost per smoker using an evidence-based proactive counseling protocol has been reported to range from $175 to $230.

Costs Associated With Operating a Quitline

- ◆ Allocate operational funding for the key activities of quitlines as follows:

    - Intake, 10% to 15%.

    - Counseling, 55% to 65%.

    - Evaluation, 10%.

    - Other, 10% to 25%.

    - Include adequate funding for evaluation in the budget calculation, as the evaluation component is critical to a quitline's success.

- ◆ Consider the following to determine how the cost of a quitline will fit into the budget for the overall tobacco control program:

    - Recruiting smokers into quitline services is likely to be substantially less expensive than recruiting them into face-to-face counseling because smokers, by a wide margin, prefer to use quitlines.

    - Increasing a quitline's budget can help meet the untapped demand for quitline services and can increase the reach of the quitline. Most statewide quitlines have, at times, experienced a greater demand for service than their staffing levels could meet.

    - In contrast, group programs often have more trained facilitators than needed for the small number of smokers attending the programs.

Promoting Quitlines

Overview

The key to a successful, cost-effective quitline media campaign is a comprehensive approach that uses a variety of media and well-crafted messages designed to reach targeted audiences. Based on the experiences of existing state quitlines, it is recommended that states work with a media professional or advertising agency with experience in social marketing to assist with the development of an effective media campaign.

This chapter covers the role of quitline promotion in the larger anti-tobacco campaign; basic concepts of traditional and social marketing that have a bearing on quitline promotion; and the use of television, radio, and other promotional channels and public relations strategies. It also includes a case study describing strategies used to promote the Arizona Smokers' Helpline.

The Media Contractor

States that have quitlines also conduct anti-tobacco media campaigns. For several reasons, the task of promoting the quitline is generally assigned to the same agency that runs the overall campaign. First, the availability of a free cessation service is just one of many messages that may need to be conveyed, and working through a single media contractor helps create a coherent campaign covering the whole range of anti-tobacco messages. This arrangement can even create synergy between campaign messages when, for example, a well-crafted ad warns about the dangers of secondhand smoke and also promotes the quitline, or when an anti-tobacco ad that does not include the quitline's phone number prepares the public for subsequent ads that do.

There are other, more basic reasons for contracting with a single agency. One is that it is easier to manage a single contract than several. Although the primary contractor may subcontract parts of the

> Working through a single media contractor helps create a coherent campaign covering the whole range of anti-tobacco messages.

campaign to other firms (for example, to one specializing in the Latino market), accountability for the success of the overall campaign remains with the primary agency.

Contracting with an agency that has social marketing expertise is also important. Social marketing differs from traditional marketing in that its goal is to promote the adoption of behaviors that will improve health or well-being, whereas the goal of traditional marketing is to sell products. Despite the difference in goals, several key concepts from traditional marketing carry over to the marketing of quitlines. States that have limited options when choosing a media contractor may want to award the entire contract to the most qualified firm it can find.

Regardless of which firm is chosen to be the media contractor for the quitline campaign, clear and frequent communication between the state, the media contractor, and the quitline is an essential component for an effective campaign. Quitline staff should be notified in advance of all media promotions. Promotional samples, press releases, proofs of print ads, on-air schedules, audiotapes of radio spots, and videotapes of TV ads should be provided before the onset of promotion. When news stories are placed with television or print media, copies of the stories should be forwarded to the quitline staff as soon as possible. Alerting them to media promotions not only helps the quitline respond to callers, but it also helps its staff gather better data on the impact of the promotion.

> Quitline staff should be notified in advance of all media promotions.

Developing the Campaign

The advertising requirements of a new quitline are different from those of existing quitlines that have name recognition and established referral systems. A new quitline must create public awareness; therefore, its campaign relies heavily on paid television and radio advertising. As awareness and referrals grow, the focus of the campaign may change: established quitlines may use advertising more to maintain a stable call volume, to target specific populations, and to pique interest on specific occasions such as the Great American Smokeout. In either case, developing a successful quitline promotional campaign is more complicated than choosing the most compelling television commercial and buying airtime. To be successful, a quitline campaign must be consumer-centered and relevant—employing the basic tenets of social marketing.

Lessons from Traditional Marketing

Social marketing differs from traditional marketing in that its goal is to promote the adoption of behaviors that will improve health or well-being, not to influence purchasing decisions. Despite the difference in goals, however, several key concepts from traditional marketing carry over to the marketing of quitlines.

One key concept is the idea that quitline services may be viewed as a kind of product. Prospective callers "buy" the product for the price of the effort to make the call. As a product, the quitline must appeal to potential buyers who wonder whether it works, how convenient it is, whether it is right for them, and so on. An effective campaign may suggest positive answers to such questions by indicating some of the benefits of using the quitline, creating demand in the process. The questions that arise in the minds of potential buyers of any product depend in large part on personal variables such as age, gender, cultural background, and socioeconomic status, so an effective campaign must start with a thorough knowledge of the target populations.

> As a product, the quitline must appeal to potential "buyers."

Another important concept is that quitline services, like all products, have a cost to the user. Potential callers foresee that they will be asked to give up an ingrained behavior, and that they will feel some discomfort in doing so. This is part of the psychological cost of calling. They may also think that the quitline staff will belittle or nag them, which adds to the perceived cost. An effective campaign may find ways to reduce this perceived cost, perhaps by suggesting that callers will find sympathy and respect, and will learn how to make quitting less painful.

A third concept is that the perceived accessibility of the product plays a part in determining whether it will be used. Since tobacco users may not know how or where to access effective cessation services, a campaign may emphasize that quitline services are "just a phone call away."

Finally, an effective quitline campaign does its marketing research up front to determine which venues—mass media channels such as television, radio, or billboards, or public relations channels such as sponsorships, participation in community events, etc.—will be most effective in reaching the target audience. Firms with ample experience developing effective social marketing campaigns for the identified target populations will not need to start from scratch, but can build on their knowledge through focus groups on quitline-specific issues with members of the target populations (Earle 2000, Weinreich 1999). It should not be assumed that an approach that worked well in one state will work equally well in another, but any information on a

Promoting Quitlines

given approach's effectiveness can be helpful as a reference point. The Centers for Disease Control and Prevention's Media Resource Center contains tobacco counter-advertisements for television, radio, print, and outdoor use that are available to the states (visit http://www.cdc.gov/tobacco/mcrc/index.htm).

Key Social Marketing Concepts

In addition to these universal marketing concepts, there are other concepts unique to social marketing that should be considered when developing a quitline campaign (Weinreich 1999). One such concept is that of primary and secondary audiences. In quitline promotion, of course, tobacco users who can be encouraged to call for service are the primary audience. But there are important secondary audiences as well. One consists of tobacco users who may not call the quitline but who will nonetheless make a quit attempt as a result of the campaign. Given the need to achieve the greatest possible reduction in the prevalence of tobacco use with limited public funds, this is a highly desirable outcome that must be a chief goal of any quitline promotional campaign.

Friends and family members of tobacco users, local tobacco control advocates, health care providers, and policy makers make up another secondary audience for quitlines. An effective marketing campaign will strive to obtain buy-in from this audience, because these individuals can help to encourage tobacco users to call. Consequently, developing partnerships with organizations that represent members of these audiences is important because these groups can help to broadcast the quitline's message to audiences that it might not otherwise reach. This is discussed more fully in Chapter 10.

Another concept is the impact of policy on behavior change. For example, creation of smoke-free restaurants and work sites may help to support the individual behaviors—calling the quitline and quitting tobacco use—that are the primary aims of a quitline campaign. In

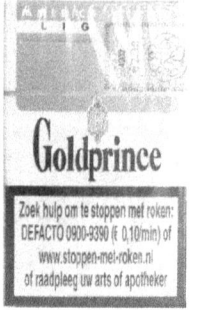

In the Netherlands, policy is being used to promote cessation in an innovative way. The European Union's new health warnings have been added to cigarette packaging, along with the telephone number for the Dutch quitline.

fact, the support works both ways, as the promulgation of effective cessation assistance makes anti-tobacco policy more universally acceptable.

A final important concept in social marketing campaigns is that, unlike campaigns selling products for profit, they do not directly pay their own way. Quitline campaigns, like many other social marketing efforts, generally depend on limited public funds that may be diverted as priorities change. For this reason, it is important to be vigilant about funding issues and to document and quantify the campaign's achievements in meeting its objectives so that a compelling case can be made to preserve its funding, if necessary.

Television and Radio

Selecting Effective Messages

Quitline media campaigns have used a wide variety of strategies, including scare tactics (such as Australia's "Every Cigarette Is Doing You Damage" campaign); heart-wrenching testimonies (such as a Massachusetts series that features people dying because they smoked); ads addressing the effects of secondhand smoke (in a California ad, a smoker laments that the life he lost was not his own, but his wife's); and humorous, sympathetic scenarios (an Arizona campaign follows a grungy "Everyman" named Chuck through the quitting process; see case study on page 79). In short, there does not appear to be any one "right" message, which may be fortunate, because a periodic change of message may help to keep the quitline fresh in the public's mind (Anderson & Zhu 2000).

> A periodic change of message may help to keep the quitline fresh in the public's mind.

On the other hand, some messages fail to attract callers (Powers 2000; Powers et al. 2000a, 2000b, 2001), or even turn them away (Rosen 2000). For example, a guilt-inducing campaign targeting pregnant smokers in Arizona caused call rates from self-identified pregnant women to decrease, relative to periods in which no such advertising was conducted. Using information from a series of focus groups, subsequent ads featured positive images of pregnant women and a message of empowerment, which significantly increased the proportion of calls from pregnant women and women of all ages (Powers et al. 2000a). States also should be aware that showing tobacco being used (for example, in ads featuring a chewer putting a dip in his mouth) could have the unintended effect of triggering tobacco use (Earle 2000), rather than the desired behavior of quitting tobacco or of calling the quitline.

Conducting formative research on media spots will provide valuable information before the spots are aired. A great deal has been learned from focus groups about what does and does not work that has considerably improved campaigns.

Determining Message Placement and Frequency

In some social marketing campaigns, the goal is to launch an issue quickly and unmistakably into the public consciousness. It may not matter if the follow-up is as strong as the launch, because the goal is to start people thinking and talking about a particular health issue. In quitline promotion, however, the main goal is to generate calls over time—enough to keep the available staff busy, but not so many that the quality of service suffers. Obtaining just the right mix of advertising to keep call volume at a steady, manageable level requires knowledge of the field.

Television and radio have been the preferred media for informing the public about quitline services and motivating large numbers of tobacco users to call. Ads can be placed in these media at predetermined times, which provides the greatest certainty that they will reach the target audience. However, this is the most expensive option. Being flexible about when the ads are aired can lower the cost of placement but may also lower the likelihood that they will reach the target populations (Weinreich 1999). Public service announcements (PSAs) are the least expensive option for television and radio but allow little targeting because the ads are generally inserted into the schedule in time slots that have not been purchased by other advertisers—often after the quitline has closed for the day. A general rule in TV and radio advertising is that sustained exposure and access to the target audience are the keys to successful media placement (Weinreich 1999).

Gross rating points and targeted ratings points are used to estimate the percentage of the target audience exposed to a message. The number and timing of the commercials are taken into account when estimating audience impact, and the cost of the buy is tied to the estimated impact. For example, commercials that air during prime time or during popular shows or special broadcasts have the potential to reach more of the target audience, but they also cost more. Because media costs are linked to gross rating points, if one time slot costs more than another, it should provide a correspondingly greater impact.

However, it is useful to remember that quitlines have a limited number of staff available to answer calls at any one time, so a large impact from one ad placement is not necessarily the goal. More frequent placements, each with a smaller impact, may be better. In this way, everyone at the quitline is kept busy and the level of customer service remains high. In general, this is easier to accomplish with radio ads than with television ads, although a television-based approach may still be needed for generating a high overall call volume.

Another way to achieve a steady call volume is by flighting, or staggering, the ads by markets or by weeks. For example, a state with multiple markets may rotate its campaign among the various markets, airing for a week in each market before moving on to the next one. Or it may air tobacco control ads in all markets at all times, and only rotate the quitline ads. Professional media buyers can help to develop a flighting plan (staggering media buys in alternating markets) that will meet the needs and budget of the state.

Other Promotional Channels

There are numerous channels for advertising besides television and radio, and while none of them is likely to have as much impact on a quitline's call volume, they have the advantage of lasting longer. These include billboards, bus signs, bus stops and kiosks, and telephone directories such as the Yellow Pages. Opportunities also exist to post promotional signs and posters in work sites, hospitals, libraries, doctors' offices, county health departments, and other locations. Besides alerting potential callers to the quitline, such efforts also help the quitline to establish a community presence. Professionally developed and graphically consistent collateral materials that can be distributed through the mail, at community events, in pharmacies, and so on, will help to solidify that presence and encourage referrals. These efforts may result in a greater number of word-of-mouth referrals each year (Anderson & Zhu 2000).

Using the media contractor to place stories in local newspapers or on TV and radio news shows is another good source of media exposure. Often called "earned media," these promotional opportunities have several advantages over paid advertising. Proactive placement of feature stories allows a quitline to work with the media to design a story for a targeted audience. Print and electronic feature stories are generally longer than news stories, allowing ample space or time to highlight the quitline's services. In addition to providing the quitline's telephone number and basic facts about its services, a feature story can share callers' personal stories. Large metropolitan areas often

> Using media relations to place stories in local newspapers or on TV and radio news shows is another good source of media exposure.

have news outlets for different populations, including foreign-language newspapers, radio stations, and television stations. There also are opportunities to highlight services in corporate newsletters, particularly those created by health insurance companies. Working with these more specialized media outlets can be an effective way to reach targeted populations. The base cost for media relations is the cost of maintaining an ambitious, well-connected media relations staff person or a public relations firm.

Also thought of as "relationship marketing," public relations activities address questions such as: What is the quitline's public image, or does it even have one? Is the quitline in the media only when there is paid advertising or when there is a crisis, or is the quitline part of the community as a whole? Relationship marketing can help establish strategies that build an organization's corporate image and community awareness of the organization. Sponsorships, memberships in community organizations, participation in community events, and volunteerism by employees are all activities that can help build relationships with work sites, health care institutions, and the general public.

Relationship marketing can also help generate referrals to the quitline. A personal referral from a trusted source, such as a friend, physician, business colleague, employer, or former quitline caller, is a powerful endorsement. Use of strategies to cultivate personal referrals has been called "viral marketing" because personal referrals spread information like a virus from one "infected" person to another. Good service infects callers with an experience that is so positive that it motivates them to tell others—creating a "buzz" about the quitline's services. This buzz can be enhanced by paid advertising, compelling media stories, and other outreach efforts.

Evaluating the Campaign

Several methods may be used to evaluate the campaign. Random-digit-dial telephone surveys can be used to estimate advertising reach (how many people remember seeing a commercial). Analysis of quitline call volume during selected ad flights or other promotions will indicate how many people took action after seeing a commercial, reading a newspaper story, or attending an event. Finally, the intake questionnaire can include a question asking callers how they heard about the quitline which will help track the effect of paid advertising as well as outreach and public relations efforts.

Arizona Ad Campaign Puts a Face on Smokers' Struggles

When the fledgling Arizona Smokers' Helpline was established in early 1995, its funding supported services for youth and pregnant women only, and the only publicity venues available were low-budget public relations and local outreach events. Consequently, the call volume was low (under 500 calls per quarter), the staff was small, and client services were limited.

In 1996, the Helpline began receiving state tobacco tax funds, and in June 1997, funding was increased to cover free cessation information, proactive telephone counseling services, and self-help publications (in Spanish and English) for all Arizonans. In January 1998, the state also began funding television advertising to promote Helpline services.

Over the next two fiscal years (1998 to 2000) the Helpline's general market advertising followed a grungy Everyman named Chuck through the stages of quitting tobacco use and beyond. These ads were aired during television prime time and, in selected spots, during the daytime soap operas. As a result of the ads, call volume increased to 500 calls per week (Powers 2000; Powers et al. 1999, 2000a, 2000b,), and the Helpline's name recognition reached 90%. In periods of high-volume advertising, as many as 75% of callers reported that they heard about the Helpline from TV.

As calls increased, client services were expanded to include relapse prevention and referrals, as well as information services on quitting and local resources, in addition to proactive counseling. During the early television campaigns, up to 95% of callers chose the Helpline's information service; however, as awareness of the Helpline increased, the percentage of clients choosing multisession proactive counseling increased to approximately 60%.

Budget constraints in fiscal years 2001 and 2002 significantly decreased television advertising, and the Helpline's recruitment strategies shifted from paid advertising to referrals. The Helpline has worked diligently with community-based tobacco control projects and health care providers to increase access to services statewide by building a network of proactive referrals to the Helpline and to community classes.

Recommendations

◆ Assign development of the quitline media campaign to a media professional or advertising agency with experience in social marketing.

◆ Use social marketing fundamentals to develop a comprehensive communication plan that identifies the quitline's multiple audiences and appropriate messages and media venues to reach those audiences.

◆ Use a variety of media and media strategies, including paid advertising and public relations.

◆ Develop, test, and implement targeted messages in appropriate venues to reach diverse populations.

◆ Coordinate all media activities with the quitline management to ensure quality customer service and appropriate staffing.

◆ Develop a consistent, recognizable graphic image and collateral materials for distribution through quitline mailings, events, work sites, health care institutions, the Internet, and other promotional venues.

Quitline Partnerships

Overview

Quitlines partner with other organizations and institutions for a number of reasons. First, funding for media campaigns is often limited, compelling states to supplement their quitline campaigns through partnerships with organizations that refer tobacco users for treatment. Even if there is funding for a robust media campaign over the short term, states often cultivate partnerships to broaden involvement, increase referrals, and sustain campaign funding. Second, community organizations participating in a state's comprehensive tobacco control program need a resource for referring people who want to quit, and quitlines partner with them to fill this need. Finally, partnership with such organizations institutionalizes the quitline in the minds of thousands of professionals across the state and makes them more likely to encourage tobacco users to quit.

Quitline partnerships range from simple affiliations that promote quitline services and stimulate referrals, to more complex affiliations intended to integrate quitlines into comprehensive tobacco control programs, to even more complex relationships with systems-level partners such as health plans. This chapter examines the range of practice in quitline partnerships, gives information about identifying and capitalizing on partnership opportunities, and provides a case study detailing efforts to create a complex network of partnerships in the state of Massachusetts.

> Quitline partnerships range from simple affiliations that promote quitline services and stimulate referrals, to more complex associations intended to integrate quitlines into comprehensive tobacco control programs.

Partnerships for Promotion and Referrals

For quitlines, the simplest and most common partnerships are those established to promote quitline services and obtain referrals. State quitlines typically form such relationships with an array of civic, community, health care, and educational groups. To help establish and maintain these partnerships, state or quitline staff may participate in events sponsored by community-based organizations or conduct

Quitline Partnerships

> ### Building Relationships with Providers
>
> The California Smoker's Helpline encourages professional inquiries from health care personnel who want to know more about the program before referring their patients. It also acknowledges physician referrals with a thank-you card and an offer of free promotional items bearing the program's name and telephone numbers. These actions have helped the Helpline develop relationships with several thousand doctors' offices around the state that actively refer patients who are interested in quitting.

onsite presentations at work sites, schools, health care facilities, or other partner sites. They may also provide promotional materials such as cards or brochures designed for members or staff of partner organizations to distribute in the field.

Start by identifying the various types of organizations that interact with the quitline's target population.

To plan and build these simple referral relationships strategically, states should start by identifying the various types of organizations that interact with the quitline's target population and that can be expected to benefit from increased awareness of quitline services, then consider which ones are likely to yield the biggest results with respect to call volume. Tapping into populations of tobacco users that have already been identified by a partner organization is a promising approach to recruitment (Lando et al. 1992).

States should consider establishing promotional relationships with a range of organizations, including health care providers, community-based organizations, colleges and universities, and other entities. Partnerships with such agencies and institutions provide distribution channels and methods to promote quitline services to a wide range of tobacco users, including underserved populations such as ethnic minority communities, new immigrants, groups targeted by the tobacco industry, and smokers who are less likely to call the quitline in response to a television or radio promotion. Simple referral and promotional relationships such as these help build a steady and predictable base of inbound calls to supplement more episodic mass media-driven call volume.

Collaborative Effort Promotes Provider Referrals

The Wisconsin Tobacco Quitline initiated a program to link health care providers to the quitline, called "FAX to Quit." Using a universal referral form, providers fax names and telephone numbers of patients who want help with cessation to the quitline, which then contacts the patients directly to provide telephone counseling.

Partnerships to Integrate the Quitline into a Comprehensive Tobacco Control Program

Although most partnerships generate referrals to the quitline, some partnerships allow quitlines to serve as gateways to other treatment options. In this way, besides providing counseling itself, a quitline can become the hub of a statewide network of cessation resources. Many state quitlines provide resource listings of local group cessation programs to all callers. Some even connect them directly to other services.

Partnerships that promote close coordination of quitline services with state, county, and local tobacco control programs are especially critical for fully integrated tobacco control programming. In states with comprehensive tobacco control programs, the quitline may be a cornerstone resource within the tobacco control infrastructure that is closely linked to all state and local initiatives and programming. For example, in New York, where the quitline works closely with local tobacco control coalitions, several of the coalitions feature the quitline in their media campaigns, and others use it as a referral resource for community-based programs serving both lay and professional communities. Quitlines can also partner with other public health and chronic disease programs and initiatives, such as cancer control, child and maternal health programs, and programs targeting pregnant women in order to promote the use of cessation services by high-risk populations.

> A quitline can become the hub of a statewide network of cessation resources.

In states with a comprehensive tobacco control program, quitlines are sometimes integrated into state or local infrastructure due to the value of their specialized expertise with tobacco cessation. In states such as Massachusetts, Arizona, Washington, and New York, quitlines are active in many statewide programs and projects. For example, in addition to providing telephone counseling services, the TryToStop

Quitline Partnerships

Tobacco Resource Center of Massachusetts plays a leading role in training, technical assistance, media campaigns, and promotional activities with state, regional, and local tobacco control programs (see case study on page 86).

> Quitlines should complement or supplement other tobacco control programming.

Quitlines should be designed to strategically complement or supplement other tobacco control programming at the state and community levels. Depending on the state's resources for cessation and its service priorities, the quitline might serve all residents or selected priority populations. Some states elect to reserve more intensive quitline services for high-priority groups, such as pregnant women or tobacco users who are uninsured or insured by Medicaid. Potential partners should be selected based on overall needs and service gaps or to help meet emerging needs, as indicated by surveillance data. For example, a quitline may work collaboratively with agencies and health care providers in communities targeted by the tobacco industry, in communities with significant health disparities, or in work sites with higher employee smoking rates, such as trade unions or metropolitan transit authorities.

Partnerships for Targeting Young Adults

Colleges and universities are natural partners for states that want to address high smoking rates among 18- to 24-year-olds. In Maryland, the American Cancer Society received a grant from the Baltimore City Health Department to provide quitline services and promote other tobacco control interventions such as Web-based initiatives on eight campuses.

Systems-Level Partnerships

States can broaden the reach of their quitlines by forming partnerships with whole systems, such as organizations with large, statewide memberships or "umbrella organizations" such as trade associations and professional societies. These types of organizations can promote quitline services or even contract for services on behalf of smaller organizations that may be difficult to reach individually.

> Health plans and health care systems are natural quitline partners.

Health plans and health care systems are natural quitline partners. Several state quitlines have established partnerships with the health plans operating in their states. In some cases, the health plans were already offering telephone counseling for tobacco cessation before the state became involved. In establishing new public quitlines, these states were careful to avoid competing with the health plans and providing a reason for them to stop offering this service. For example, before Minnesota established its quitline, various health plans, most notably Blue Cross/Blue Shield of Minnesota and the Mayo Clinic, were already providing telephone counseling for their members, who represented the majority of Minnesotans. Likewise, when Utah established its adult quitline, Intermountain Health Care was already offering telephone counseling services that covered over a fifth of state residents. Under partnership agreements with the statewide quitlines, each of these plans still provide their members with cessation counseling. The statewide quitline helps enroll plan members into services by assessing all callers for insurance coverage and transferring members to the appropriate plan.

Other states have also developed innovative partnerships with health plans. Massachusetts negotiated with all of its major health plans to adopt a universal system of fax referral and proactive telephone counseling (see case study on page 86). The Roswell Park Quitline (New York State), in partnership with Univera Healthcare, developed a fee-for-service counseling program, called QUIT123, for high-risk members of the health plan. The plan pays for a quitline service that allows physicians' offices to fax a patient referral form to the quitline. Quitline staff then proactively contact the patient for counseling. A patient feedback form is then sent to the referring physician. The quitline also provides this service to other health care providers.

States have explored other cost-sharing ideas for partnership with health plans as a way of expanding the reach of their quitlines. Where practical, quitlines should build partnerships, with linkages and reinforcements, at all levels of the health care system. For example, proactive patient contact via fax referral and feedback reports from the quitline can both be used to reinforce interventions with providers and partner organizations. Collaboration among the major health plans to build and promote a universal system of referral to statewide quitline services is ideal. For providers—especially those who participate in many health plans—such a system can reduce barriers to access to effective treatment for their patients. Obtaining endorsements from and conducting joint promotions with medical and professional societies and voluntary organizations through their member newsletters, Web sites, and annual meetings are other ways to encourage and reinforce the use of quitline services.

> Where practical, quitlines should build partnerships, with linkages and reinforcements, at all levels of the health care system.

Quitline Partnerships

QuitWorks—Massachusetts Partnership Links 12,000 Providers and Their Patients to Proactive Telephone Counseling

QuitWorks is an unparalleled partnership between the Massachusetts Department of Public Health and eight commercial and Medicaid health plans in the state. QuitWorks links health care providers and their patients who smoke to proactive telephone counseling and to other tobacco treatment services. Launched in 2002 with 6,000 primary care providers, the QuitWorks program has been extended to medical specialists, dentists, and health plan case managers. It has also been adapted for use in hospitals and community health centers and supports systems-level changes in these settings. (See Chapter 11 for additional information on system-level changes.)

Central to QuitWorks is a universally endorsed fax enrollment form that can be used by any provider with any patient, regardless of health insurance status. Patients enrolled in QuitWorks are called by the TryToStop Tobacco Resource Center and offered free multisession proactive counseling, Internet counseling at http://www.trytostop.org, and referral to community-based treatment programs. Physicians receive feedback reports on patient progress and outcomes, and the health plans, hospitals, and health centers receive customized quarterly aggregate reports.

All physicians in Massachusetts have access to a QuitWorks kit that contains office systems tools, patient enrollment forms, and patient education materials. Kits have been delivered to provider practices by more than 100 health plan provider representatives who were trained by the University of Massachusetts Medical School. QuitWorks materials are also available online at http://www.quitworks.org.

In institutional settings, a QuitWorks team works with hospital quality improvement and clinical leadership to integrate QuitWorks into patient care systems, customize enrollment and consent forms, and train clinicians. To date, more than 5,000 practices and providers in Massachusetts have received QuitWorks kits, and thousands of smokers have used QuitWorks services.

By working together with the state, Massachusetts health plans are helping to improve access for all patients to evidence-based tobacco treatment. The Massachusetts Medical Society, Massachusetts Dental Society, Massachusetts Academy of Pediatrics, American Cancer Society, American Heart Association, American Lung Association, and Massachusetts League of Community Health Centers also support the QuitWorks program.

Recommendations

- Explore opportunities to partner with health care systems, community groups, and business and professional organizations to promote quitline services.

- Target whole systems such as health plans, educational systems, public health and human service agencies, insurers, business and trade associations, and other organizations likely to have large memberships.

- Establish relationships that promote close coordination of quitline services with state, county, and local tobacco control programs.

- Select partners and target populations strategically and in alignment with overall tobacco control program goals, needs, and priority populations.

- Form partnerships designed to promote quitline services and encourage systems-level interventions and policy changes within partner organizations.

Future Directions

Overview

Future developments in quitlines will likely occur in two main areas. First, the menu of services they offer will expand to include new counseling protocols for special populations and intervention strategies that go beyond counseling. Second, quitlines will increase their population impact as their current partnerships become better established and new opportunities for collaboration and provision of specialized services appear. Helping to drive these changes will be increased efforts among people in different states to provide mutual assistance with protocol development, operations management, and program evaluation.

Increasing the Menu of Services

Although research has shown telephone counseling to be effective in various settings, the evidence thus far has been limited to English- and Spanish-speaking adult smokers. As evidence becomes available on effective interventions for other populations, and as quitlines expand their capacity to provide culturally sensitive and language-specific services to more communities, the menu of evidence-based counseling services will broaden.

> As evidence becomes available on effective interventions for other populations, the menu of evidence-based counseling services will broaden.

Meanwhile, as quitlines accumulate clinical experience and respond to new challenges, they will make adjustments to their existing protocols. For example, smokers using newly developed pharmacotherapies may require different counseling schedules. Because each medical regimen has its own time frame, quitlines will need to adjust their protocols to support patients using these medications, assess their status at the end of the medication regimen, and help them as they transition off the medications to reduce the risk of relapse.

As quitlines become more institutionalized within their states, the number of repeat callers will grow, increasing the need for effective ways to help them. At the same time, the number of former callers

> The ever-increasing number of former callers who have not yet quit for good will induce quitlines to find ways to help them move forward.

Future Directions

> As quitlines attempt to stretch their resources as far as possible, they will begin adopting intervention strategies to supplement mailed materials and telephone counseling.

who relapse but never call back will also grow, which will induce quitline operators to find ways to help them move forward. The familiarity these former callers have with quitlines will present opportunities for reconnection, allowing quitline staff to help them build on their past quit attempts. Proactive protocols may prove especially effective with these smokers.

As quitlines attempt to stretch their resources as far as possible, they will begin adopting intervention strategies to supplement self-help materials and telephone counseling. Strategies that would entail significant start-up costs but low marginal costs include Web-based activities, interactive voice response (IVR) services, and tailored mailings.

For example, as the proportion of people using the Internet increases, its potential as a medium for tailored cessation assistance also increases. It may be possible to direct some callers to a Web-based relapse prevention module in lieu of follow-up counseling, although this strategy has not yet been tested. Likewise, the proliferation of IVR services, through which callers access detailed and personalized information, raises the possibility of providing cessation information through this medium. Finally, the lower-tech but more widely applicable method of sending automatically generated tailored letters may enable quitlines to increase their level of engagement with callers to better support their efforts to quit. However, all of these innovative strategies would need to be evaluated before widespread use could be recommended.

Combinations of intervention strategies, whether current or emerging, may be managed using customer relationship management (CRM) software. This software is intended to make it feasible for organizations to serve a diverse clientele through a range of media (telephone, fax, e-mail, etc.) according to each individual client's preference. Although existing CRM applications have had limited success in helping organizations achieve this goal, refinements are ongoing, and quitlines may come to rely on such programs as their intervention strategies become more complex.

Increasing the Population Impact

States that have established comprehensive tobacco control programs face difficult choices as they balance priorities. The question of how much funding to devote to cessation, as opposed to other priorities, such as preventing youth access to tobacco or reducing exposure to secondhand smoke, is not easy to answer. Therefore, it is incumbent on those who work on the cessation side of tobacco control to ensure that their efforts are not only effective at the level of individual tobacco users, but also have as big an impact as possible at the population level.

Quitlines have gained prominence because they have provided evidence of their clinical efficacy as well as their effectiveness in real-world settings, and because of their potential to make cessation services more universally available. However, research is still needed on the effect of the promotion and utilization of quitlines on the prevalence of tobacco use in states that have them.

Every existing quitline serves thousands of tobacco users per year—a volume rarely achieved by other behavioral services—and many quitlines have seen dramatic increases in usage over time. Even so, quitlines currently reach only 1% to 5% of the tobacco users in their states per year. Therefore, to have a more substantial population impact, utilization rates must increase even further. It has been suggested, based on the experience of private quitlines serving health plans, that statewide quitlines could potentially reach 15% of the tobacco-using population per year (McAfee 2002).

Partnering for Growth

The rate at which quitlines are utilized appears to be limited not by a lack of interest in quitting or by a belief that help is not needed (Zhu & Anderson 2000), but by the level of funding available for promotion and operations. The large spikes in call volume commonly experienced during promotional campaigns also indicate a large untapped demand for services. Consequently, as quitlines try to increase their population impact, they will look for new ways to increase public awareness and the use of services and new ways to pay for those services.

> The large spikes in call volume commonly experienced during promotional campaigns indicate a large untapped demand for services.

One potential way for quitlines to accomplish both objectives is by partnering more fully with the health care system. About 70% of smokers visit their physicians at least once a year (CDC 1993a), but fewer than 5% have used a quitline (Zhu 2002a). As mentioned in Chapter 1, time constraints often prevent physicians from providing personal cessation counseling to their tobacco-using patients. Physicians can circumvent this barrier by referring these patients to a quitline (Schroeder 2003). Many state quitlines already work with physicians, but their collaboration tends to be limited to individual physicians who have a particular interest in cessation.

Future Directions

To dramatically increase health care-initiated utilization, quitline referrals must be instituted on a systems level. If clinics regularly identified tobacco users, advised them to quit, and obtained their consent to be contacted by a cessation specialist, quitline staff could proactively call them to provide counseling. Efforts in this area have already begun. In Arizona, for example, the quitline uses faxed referrals to identify clients from the Special Supplemental Nutrition Program for Women, Infants, and Children (WIC) to receive a proactive call. WIC identifies clients who smoke, obtains their written permission to have the quitline contact them to assist with smoking cessation, and faxes the referral to the quitline. Studies have shown that a proactive approach can dramatically increase the percentage of tobacco-using patients receiving cessation counseling. In one study, counseling utilization rates were increased from 3% to 35% through this approach (Cummins et al. 2002).

A system that allows clinic staff to enroll a patient (with his or her consent) into counseling by logging onto a secure Internet-based scheduling system while the patient is still in the doctor's office could make the referral process even more efficient. A cost-sharing model in which managed care organizations (MCOs) pay only for services directly attributable to this scheduling system, while the state continues to pay for all other services received, would demonstrate effective partnering between the public and private sectors and dramatically increase both the reach of quitlines and the treatment of tobacco-related disease.

It is worth noting that such collaboration between quitlines and MCOs could also improve the quality of treatment of tobacco dependence within the health care system. For example, quitlines could enhance patient compliance with physician-prescribed cessation treatments such as nicotine replacement therapy by providing patients with detailed information about its proper use, answers to questions about side effects, and so forth. Quitlines could even dispense quitting aids directly, removing barriers to access and addressing patients' ambivalence about following through with their physicians' recommendations. Some quitlines are already doing this (McAfee 2002), as studies have shown that reducing the burden of obtaining pharmacotherapies increases their usage (Hopkins et al. 2001).

> A quitline could serve as the hub of a comprehensive statewide system of evidence-based cessation services.

Quitlines also could support patient compliance with cessation treatments by helping them access other support systems available locally (e.g., culturally specific cessation classes), either alone or in combination with quitline counseling. In this way, a quitline could serve as the hub of a comprehensive statewide system of evidence-based cessation services. It would then increase its population impact not only by providing effective counseling services, but also by enhancing the use of other available cessation resources, including pharmacotherapies and community cessation programs (Pacific Center on Health and Tobacco 2003).

As states work to broaden the reach of their quitlines, they must address the disproportionate burden borne by certain groups of tobacco users. They should not be content merely to increase overall utilization rates. They must also help address disparities in the prevalence of tobacco use and utilization of cessation resources. Quitlines have already been shown to reach more tobacco users of ethnic minority backgrounds than do traditional clinic-based programs (Zhu et al. 1995). With smoking increasingly concentrated among people of low socioeconomic status (SES), it is imperative that quitlines increase their efforts to help this segment of the population. Many low-SES tobacco users have inadequate medical insurance and do not use the health care system as frequently as others. Quitlines have functioned as "equalizers" in the field of cessation assistance because telephones are among the few things that most people own regardless of SES (Fiore et al. 2004). In addition, state quitline services are provided at no cost to callers. These two considerations make quitlines ideal for community-wide intervention in low-SES areas. For example, targeted billboard campaigns can be waged in ZIP code areas of low SES.

> States must also address disparities in the prevalence of tobacco use and utilization of cessation resources.

The goal of increasing the population impact of quitlines could be strongly supported by policies such as those recommended by the Cessation Subcommittee of the U.S. Department of Health and Human Services' Interagency Committee on Smoking and Health (Fiore et al. 2004). In its National Action Plan for Tobacco Cessation, this federal advisory committee called for the establishment of a federally funded national network of quitlines that would provide universal access to evidence-based counseling and medications for tobacco cessation and a national portal to state or regionally managed quitlines. It also called for a level of financial support far exceeding what quitlines currently receive.

To help advance supportive policies, quitlines must consolidate their achievements and establish their value as an effective population-based approach to cessation. Continuing research and development are also needed to provide more comprehensive scientific support for such policies.

> To help advance supportive policies, quitlines must establish their value as an effective population-based approach to cessation.

Increasing Cooperation

With the goals of helping the field to consolidate its achievements and taking a more active role in reducing the prevalence of tobacco use in their states, quitline funders, researchers, and operators have formed a consortium to improve cooperation among states with quitlines (Ossip-Klein 2002, Bailey 2003). The consortium is intended not only to help the member organizations, but also to help advance the field itself.

Several important benefits should result from this type of collaboration. First, a consortium allows data and experience to be shared more efficiently and completely than is usually the case with the standard publication process. For example, practical information concerning quitline operations that is unlikely to be published in peer-reviewed journals can easily be disseminated through a consortium. Second, a consortium facilitates collaboration on research and education. Natural variations that exist among quitlines provide ideal opportunities for research. They also induce a need for the ongoing accumulation and quick dissemination of knowledge among quitline funders and practitioners. Third, a consortium can set minimum standards for service and promote appropriate quality assurance measures to ensure that member quitlines operate from a strong evidence base. Finally, a consortium can improve public and policy awareness of what quitlines can and should do to help reduce the prevalence of tobacco use.

References

Anderson CM, Zhu SH. The California Smokers' Helpline and low-SES smokers. Paper presented at the National Conference on Tobacco or Health, San Francisco, CA, November 19–21, 2002.

Anderson CM, Zhu SH. *The California Smokers' Helpline: A Case Study.* Sacramento, CA: California Department of Health Services, 2000.

Bailey L. The alliance for tobacco cessation: lessons learned about expanding coverage for evidence-based tobacco dependence treatment. Paper presented at the Ninth Annual Meeting of the Society for Research on Nicotine and Tobacco, New Orleans, LA, February 19–22, 2003.

Borland R, Balmford J, Hunt D. The effectiveness of personally tailored computer-generated advice letters for smoking cessation. *Addiction* 2004;99(3):369–377.

Borland R, Segan CJ, Livingston PM, Owen N. The effectiveness of callback counselling for smoking cessation: a randomized trial. *Addiction* 2001;96(6):881–889.

Burns DM. Smoking cessation: recent indicators of what's working at a population level. In: National Cancer Institute. *Population Based Smoking Cessation: Proceedings of a Conference on What Works to Influence Cessation in the General Population.* Smoking and Tobacco Control Monograph No. 12. Bethesda, MD: U.S. Department of Health and Human Services, National Institutes of Health, National Cancer Institute, NIH Pub. No. 00-4892, November 2000:99–128.

Centers for Disease Control and Prevention, Office on Smoking and Health. Unpublished quitline data.

Centers for Disease Control and Prevention. Annual smoking-attributable mortality, years of potential life lost, and economic costs—United States, 1995–1999. *Morbidity and Mortality Weekly Report* 2002a;51(14):300–303.

Centers for Disease Control and Prevention. Cigarette smoking among adults—United States, 2000. *Morbidity and Mortality Weekly Report* 2002b;51(29):642–645.

Centers for Disease Control and Prevention. *Best Practices for Comprehensive Tobacco Control Programs—August 1999.* Atlanta, GA: U.S. Department of Health and Human Services, Centers for Disease Control and Prevention, National Center for Chronic Disease Prevention and Health Promotion, Office on Smoking and Health, 1999.

References

Centers for Disease Control and Prevention. Physician and other health-care professional counseling of smokers to quit—United States, 1991. *Morbidity and Mortality Weekly Report* 1993a;42(44);854–857.

Centers for Disease Control and Prevention. Use of smokeless tobacco among adults—United States, 1991. *Morbidity and Mortality Weekly Report* 1993b;42(14):263–266.

Cummins SE, Zhu SH, Anderson CM. Telephone quitlines for high-risk or hard-to-reach populations. Paper presented at the National Conference on Tobacco or Health, San Francisco, CA, November 19–21, 2002.

Curry S, McBride C, Grothaus LC, et al. A randomized trial of self-help materials, personalized feedback, and telephone counseling with nonvolunteer smokers. *Journal of Consulting and Clinical Psychology* 1995;63(6):1005–1014.

Earle R. *The Art of Cause Marketing: How to Use Advertising to Change Personal Behavior and Public Policy.* Lincolnwood, IL: NTC Business Books, 2000.

Farrelly MC, Pechacek TF, Chaloupka FJ. The impact of tobacco control program expenditures on aggregate cigarette sales: 1981–2000. *Journal of Health Economics* 2003;22(5):843–859.

Fiore MC, Croyle RT, Curry SJ, et al. Preventing 3 million premature deaths and helping 5 million smokers quit: a national action plan for tobacco cessation. *American Journal of Public Health* 2004;94(2):205–210.

Fiore MC, Bailey WC, Cohen SJ, et al. *Treating Tobacco Use and Dependence.* Clinical Practice Guideline. Rockville, MD: U.S. Department of Health and Human Services, Public Health Services, June 2000.

Fishbein HA, Unger JB, Johnson CA, et al. Interaction of population-based approaches for tobacco control. In: National Cancer Institute. *Population Based Smoking Cessation: Proceedings of a Conference on What Works to Influence Cessation in the General Population.* Smoking and Tobacco Control Monograph No. 12. Bethesda, MD: U.S. Department of Health and Human Services, National Institutes of Health, National Cancer Institute, NIH Pub. No. 00-4892, November 2000:223–233.

Flay BR. Efficacy and effectiveness trials (and other phases of research) in the development of health promotion programs. *Preventive Medicine* 1986;15(5):451–474.

Floyd RL, Rimer BK, Giovino GA, et al. A review of smoking in pregnancy: effects on pregnancy outcomes and cessation efforts. *Annual Review of Public Health* 1993;14:379–411.

Greenwald P, Cullen JW. The new emphasis in cancer control. *Journal of the National Cancer Institute* 1985;74(3):543–551.

Hatsukami DK, Severson HH. Oral spit tobacco: addiction, prevention and treatment. *Nicotine & Tobacco Research* 1999;1(1):21–44.

Hollis J, Polen M, Whitlock E, et al. Efficacy of a brief tobacco prevention and cessation program for teens seen in routine medical care (Teen REACH). Paper presented at the National Cancer Institute Youth Tobacco Research Meeting, Palm Harbor, FL, June 2002.

Hopkins DP, Briss PA, Ricard CJ, et al. Reviews of evidence regarding interventions to reduce tobacco use and exposure to environmental tobacco smoke. *American Journal of Preventive Medicine* 2001;20(Suppl 2):16–66.

Hughes JR, Keely JP, Niaura RS, et al. Measures of abstinence in clinical trials: issues and recommendations. *Nicotine & Tobacco Research* 2003;5(1):13–25.

Lando HA, Hellerstedt WL, Pirie PL, et al. Brief supportive telephone outreach as a recruitment and intervention strategy for smoking cessation. *American Journal of Public Health* 1992;82(1):41–46.

Lichtenstein E, Glasgow RE. Smoking cessation: what have we learned over the past decade? *Journal of Consulting and Clinical Psychology* 1992;60(4):518–527.

Lichtenstein E, Zhu SH, McAfee T. Smoking cessation quitlines: fusing research and practice. Symposium presented at the 24th Annual Meeting of the Society for Behavioral Medicine, Salt Lake City, UT, March 19–22, 2003.

Lichtenstein E, Glasgow RE, Lando HA, et al. Telephone counseling for smoking cessation: rationales and meta-analytic review of evidence. *Health Education Research* 1996;11(2):243–257.

McAfee T. Increasing the population impact of quitlines. Paper presented at the North American Quitline Conference, Phoenix, AZ, May 8–10, 2002.

McAfee T, Sofian NS, Wilson J, et al. The role of tobacco intervention in population-based health care: a case study. *American Journal of Preventive Medicine* 1998;14(Suppl 3):46–52.

McAlister AL, Rabius V, Geiger A, et al. Telephone assistance for smoking cessation: one year cost effectiveness estimations. *Tobacco Control* 2004;13(1):85–86.

McDonald P, Colwell B, Backinger CL, et al. Better practices for youth tobacco cessation: evidence of review panel. *American Journal of Health Behavior* 2003;27(Suppl 2):S144–S158.

Melvin CL, Dolan-Mullen P, Windsor RA, et al. Recommended cessation counselling for pregnant women who smoke: a review of the evidence. *Tobacco Control* 2000;9(Suppl III):iii80–iii84.

Mermelstein R. Youth smoking cessation. Paper presented at Tobacco Control Research: Investing in Science for the Public's Health. Washington, DC, June 17–19, 2003.

Niaura R, Abrams DB. Smoking cessation: progress, priorities, and prospectus. *Journal of Consulting and Clinical Psychology* 2002;70(3):494–509.

New Jersey Comprehensive Tobacco Control Program. *2001 Annual Report*. New Jersey Department of Health and Senior Services, 2001. Available at http://www.state.nj.us/health/as/ctcp/annualreport.htm. Accessed March 24, 2004.

References

Orleans CT, Melvin CL, Marx JF, et al. National action plan to reduce smoking during pregnancy: the National Partnership to Help Pregnant Smokers Quit. *Nicotine & Tobacco Research* 2004; 6(Suppl 2):S269–S277.

Orleans CT, Schoenbach VJ, Wagner EH, et al. Self-help quit smoking interventions: effects of self-help materials, social support instructions, and telephone counseling. *Journal of Consulting and Clinical Psychology* 1991;59(3):439–448.

Ossip-Klein DJ. The concept of a consortium for quitlines. Paper presented at the North American Quitline Conference, Phoenix, AZ, May 8–10, 2002.

Ossip-Klein DJ, McIntosh S. Quitlines in North America: evidence base and applications. *American Journal of Medical Science* 2003;326(4):201–205.

Ossip-Klein DJ, Giovino GA, Megahed N, et al. Effects of a smoker's hotline: results of a 10-county self-help trial. *Journal of Consulting and Clinical Psychology* 1991;59(2):325–332.

Owen L. Impact of a telephone helpline for smokers who called during a mass media campaign. *Tobacco Control* 2000;9(2):148–154.

Pacific Center on Health and Tobacco. Linking a Network: Integrating Quitlines with Health Care Systems, 2003. Available at http://www.paccenter.org. Accessed March 24, 2004.

Padgett DI, Zhu SH, Sun J, Strychacz C. Characteristics of smokeless tobacco users calling a statewide tobacco cessation quitline. Paper presented at the National Conference on Tobacco or Health, San Francisco, CA, November 19–21, 2002.

Peto R, Darby S, Deo H, et al. Smoking, smoking cessation, and lung cancer in the UK since 1950: combination of national statistics with two case-control studies. *British Medical Journal* 2000;321(7257):323–329.

Powers P. Impact of media on the Arizona Smokers' Helpline: three-year comparison. 11th World Conference on Tobacco or Health, Chicago, August 6–11, 2000. Available at http://www.tepp.org/presentations. Accessed March 24, 2004.

Powers P, Wentzel TM, Ranger-Moore J. Impact of pharmacotherapy usage and social support on quit rates for Hispanic clients of the Arizona Smokers' Helpline. Paper presented at the National Conference on Tobacco or Health, New Orleans, LA, November 27–29, 2001. Available at http://128.196.174.132/bigfiles/hispanics-NCTOH2001.ppt. Accessed March 24, 2004.

Powers P, Wentzel TM, Ranger-Moore J, et al. Attracting motivated quitters to a smokers' helpline using television advertising. Poster presented at the 21st Annual Meeting of the Society for Behavioral Medicine, Nashville, TN, April 5–8, 2000a. Available at http://www.tepp.org/presentations/chuck2000/index.htm. Accessed March 24, 2004.

Powers P, Ranger-Moore J, Wentzel TM, et al. Impact of television advertising on helpline clients' stages of change. Poster presented at the Sixth Annual Meeting of the Society for Research on Nicotine and Tobacco, Arlington, VA, February 18–20, 2000b. Available at http://www.tepp.org/presentations/Impact_2000/index.htm. Accessed March 24, 2004.

Powers P, Wentzel TM, Ranger-Moore J, et al. Effects of television advertising on tobacco use cessation helpline calls. Poster presented at the 127th Annual Meeting of the American Public Health Association, Chicago, November 7–11, 1999.

Rosen E. *The Anatomy of Buzz* New York: Doubleday, 2000.

Schroeder SA. Thirty seconds to save a life: what busy clinicians can do to help their patients quit smoking. Presented at a meeting of BlueCross/BlueShield Association executives, San Francisco, CA, November 12, 2003. Available at http://smokingcessationleadership.ucsf.edu. Accessed April 10, 2004.

Severson HH, Andrews JA, Lichtenstein E, et al. A self-help cessation program for smokeless tobacco users: comparison of two interventions. *Nicotine & Tobacco Research* 2000;2(4):363–370.

Stead LF, Lancaster T, Perera R. Telephone counselling for smoking cessation (Cochrane Review). In: *The Cochrane Library 2004*, Issue 1. Chichester, UK: John Wiley & Sons, Ltd, 2004.

Stevens C. Designing an effective counteradvertising campaign—California. *Cancer* 1998;83 (Suppl 12):2736–2741.

Stevens VJ, Glasgow RE, Hollis JF, Mount K. Implementation and effectiveness of a brief smoking-cessation intervention for hospital patients. *Medical Care* 2000;38(5):451–459.

Swan GE, McAfee T, Curry SJ, et al. Effectiveness of bupropion sustained release for smoking cessation in a health care setting: a randomized trial. *Archives of Internal Medicine* 2003;163(19):2337–2344.

Taylor DH, Hasselblad V, Henley SJ, et al. Benefits of smoking cessation for longevity. *American Journal of Public Health* 2002;92(6):990–996.

U.S. Department of Health and Human Services. *Healthy People 2010.* 2nd ed. With Understanding and Improving Health and Objectives for Improving Health. 2 vols. Washington, DC: U.S. Department of Health and Human Services, 2000a.

U.S. Department of Health and Human Services. *Reducing Tobacco Use: A Report of the Surgeon General.* Atlanta, GA: U.S. Department of Health and Human Services, Centers for Disease Control and Prevention, Office on Smoking and Health, 2000b.

U.S. Department of Health and Human Services. *Tobacco Use Among U.S. Racial/Ethnic Minority Groups—African Americans, American Indians and Alaska Natives, Asian Americans and Pacific Islanders, and Hispanics: A Report of the Surgeon General.* Atlanta, GA: U.S. Department of Health and Human Services, Centers for Disease Control and Prevention, National Center for Chronic Disease Prevention and Health Promotion, Office on Smoking and Health, 1998.

Velicer WF, Prochaska JO, Rossi JS, Snow MG. Assessing outcome in smoking cessation studies. *Psychological Bulletin* 1992;111(1):23–41.

Waa A, Glasgow H, McCulloch M. Subsidisation of nicotine replacement therapies through the New Zealand Quitline. Paper presented at the Second European Quitline Conference, Barcelona, Spain, September 6–8, 2000.

References

Wakefield M, Borland R. Saved by the bell: the role of telephone helpline services in the context of mass-media anti-smoking campaigns. *Tobacco Control* 2000;9(2):117–119.

Weinreich NK. *Hands-On Social Marketing*. Thousand Oaks, CA: Sage Publications, 1999.

Zhu SH. A quitline for teen smokers. Paper presented at the Youth Tobacco Research Meeting, Washington, DC, June 17–19, 2003.

Zhu SH. A survey of quitlines in North America. Paper presented at the North America Quitline Conference, Phoenix, AZ, May 8–10, 2002a.

Zhu SH. Special populations: adolescents, pregnant women, SLT users. Paper presented at the North American Quitline Conference, Phoenix, AZ, May 8–10, 2002b.

Zhu SH. Telephone quitlines for smoking cessation. In: National Cancer Institute. *Population Based Smoking Cessation: Proceedings of a Conference on What Works to Influence Cessation in the General Population*. Smoking and Tobacco Control Monograph No. 12. Bethesda, MD: U.S. Department of Health and Human Services, National Institutes of Health, National Cancer Institute, NIH Pub. No. 00–4892, November 2000:189–198.

Zhu SH, Anderson CM, Johnson CE, et al. A centralized telephone service for tobacco cessation: the California experience. *Tobacco Control* 2000;9(Suppl II):ii48–ii55.

Zhu SH, Anderson CM. Bridging the clinical and public health approaches to smoking cessation: California Smokers' Helpline. In: Jamner MS, Stokols D, eds. *Promoting Human Wellness: New Frontiers for Research, Practice, and Policy*. Berkeley, CA: University of California Press, 2000:378–394.

Zhu SH, Anderson CM, Tedeschi GJ, et al. Evidence of real-world effectiveness of a telephone quitline for smokers. *New England Journal of Medicine* 2002;347:1087–1093.

Zhu SH, Stretch V, Balabanis M, et al. Telephone counseling for smoking cessation: effects of single-session and multiple-session interventions. *Journal of Consulting and Clinical Psychology* 1996;64(1):202–211.

Zhu SH, Rosbrook B, Anderson CM, et al. The demographics of help-seeking for smoking cessation in California and the role of the California Smokers' Helpline. *Tobacco Control* 1995;4(Suppl I): S9–S15.

Appendixes

Appendix A: State Quitline Information[†]

State (Adult Smoking Prevalence*)	Date Service Began	Language Services[††]	Primary Contractor	Quitline Contact Information
Alaska (29.4%)	January 2002	None	Providence Alaska Medical Center	1-888-842-QUIT (7848)
Arizona (23.5%)	January 1995	Spanish	University of Arizona	1-800-556-6222 E-mail: ashline1@u.arizona.edu http://www.ashline.org
Arkansas (26.3%)	January 2003	Spanish	Mayo Clinic Foundation	1-866-NOW-QUIT (669-7848) http://www.stampoutsmoking.com
California (16.4%)	August 1992	Cantonese, Korean, Mandarin, Spanish, Vietnamese	University of California, San Diego	1-800-NO-BUTTS (672-8887) 1-800-45-NO-FUME (456-6386) (Spanish) 1-800-838-8917 (Mandarin & Cantonese) 1-800-778-8440 (Vietnamese) 1-800-556-5564 (Korean) 1-800-844-CHEW (2439) (Smokeless) TDD: 1-800-933-4833 E-mail: cshoutreach@ucsd.edu http://www.californiasmokershelpline.org
Colorado (20.4%)	October 2001	Spanish	National Jewish Medical and Research Center	1-800-639-QUIT (7848) TTY: 1-800-659-2656 http://www.co.quitnet.com
Connecticut (19.5%)	November 2001	Spanish, Telephone Translation Service	United Way of Connecticut Infoline in partnership with Hartford Hospital	1-866-END-HABIT (363-4224) E-mail: quitline@ctunitedway.org http://www.ctquitline.org
Delaware (24.7%)	February 2001	Spanish, AT&T Language Line	American Cancer Society	1-866-409-1858 http://www.state.de.us/dhss/dph/dpc/quitline.html
District of Columbia (20.4%)	December 2003	Spanish	American Legacy Foundation	1-800-399-5589 http://www.americanlegacy.org
Florida (22.1%)	December 2001	Spanish, Haitian-Creole	American Cancer Society	1-877-U-CAN-NOW (822-6669) TTY: 1-866-228-4327
Georgia (23.3%)	September 2001	Spanish, AT&T Language Line	Center for Health Promotion, Inc.	1-877-270-STOP (7867) 1-877-2NO-FUME (266-3863) (Spanish) TTY: 1-877-777-6534 E-mail: gatups@aol.com http://www.unitegeorgia.com/resources/

† Compiled by Center for Tobacco Cessation, updated December 2003.
Telephone numbers and Web sites are subject to change without notice.

* Estimates of current adult smoking prevalence for each state are from the 2002 Behavioral Risk Factor Surveillance System. Centers for Disease Control and Prevention. State-specific prevalence of current cigarette smoking among adults, and policies and attitudes about secondhand smoke—United States, 2002. *Morbidity and Mortality Weekly Report* 2004;52(53):1277–1280.

†† In addition to English.

Appendix A: State Quitline Information[†]

State (Adult Smoking Prevalence*)	Date Service Began	Language Services[††]	Primary Contractor	Quitline Contact Information
Illinois (22.9%)	1999	Spanish	American Lung Association	1-866-QUIT-YES (784-8937) http://www.idph.state.il.us/TobaccoWebSite/quitsmoking.htm
Iowa (23.1%)	May 2001	Spanish	University of Iowa, Iowa Tobacco Research Center	1-866-U-CAN-TRY (822-6879) http://www.quitlineiowa.org
Kansas (22.1%)	October 2003	Spanish, Vietnamese	Wellplace (Pioneer Behavioral Health)	1-866-KAN-STOP (526-7867)
Louisiana (23.9%)	1999	N/A	Tobacco Control Resource Center	1-800-LUNG-USA (586-4872)
Maine (23.6%)	August 2001	None	Center for Tobacco Independence	1-800-207-1230 TTY: 1-800-457-1220
Massachusetts (19.0%)	July 1994	Portuguese, Spanish, AT&T Language Line	JSI Research and Training Institute, Inc.	1-800-TRY-TO-STOP (879-8678) 1-800-8-DEJALO (833-5256) TDD: 1-800-833-1477 E-mail: trytostop@trytostop.org http://www.trytostop.org
Michigan (24.2%)	October 2003	None	Leade Health	1-800-480-7848
Minnesota (21.7%)	April 2001	Spanish, AT&T Language Line	Center for Health Promotion, Inc.	1-877-270-STOP (7867) 1-877-2NO-FUME (266-3863) (Spanish) TTY: 1-877-777-6534 http://www.mpaat.org
Mississippi (27.4%)	September 1999	Spanish	Information and Quality Healthcare	1-800-244-9100 1-877-487-2228 http://www.quitlinems.com
Nebraska (22.8%)	June 2002	Korean, Spanish, Vietnamese	Wellplace (Pioneer Development and Support)	1-866-632-7848
Nevada (26.0%)	2001	Spanish, Tagalog	University of Nevada School of Medicine	1-888-866-6642 702-877-0684 (Las Vegas only)

† Compiled by Center for Tobacco Cessation, updated December 2003.
Telephone numbers and Web sites are subject to change without notice.

* Estimates of current adult smoking prevalence for each state are from the 2002 Behavioral Risk Factor Surveillance System. Centers for Disease Control and Prevention. State-specific prevalence of current cigarette smoking among adults, and policies and attitudes about secondhand smoke—United States, 2002. *Morbidity and Mortality Weekly Report* 2004;52(53):1277–1280.

†† In addition to English.

Appendix A: State Quitline Information[†]

State (Adult Smoking Prevalence*)	Date Service Began	Language Services[††]	Primary Contractor	Quitline Contact Information
New Hampshire (23.2%)	August 2002	Portuguese, Spanish, AT&T Language Line	JSI Research and Training Institute, Inc.	1-800-TRY-TO-STOP 1-800-8-DEJALO (833-5256) TDD: 1-800-833-1477 E-mail: trytostop@trytostop.org http://www.trytostop.org
New Jersey (19.1%)	October 1999	Spanish, AT&T Language Line	Mayo Clinic	1-866-NJSTOPS TTY: 1-866-257-2971 http://www.nj.quitnet.com
New Mexico (21.2%)	January 2001	Spanish	NCI's Cancer Information Service	1-877-44U-QUIT http://www.thestink.org
New York (22.4%)	January 2000	AT&T Language Line	Roswell Park Cancer Institute	1-866-NY-QUITS (697-8487) TTY: 1-800-280-1213 1-866-293-1796 (New York City Medicaid) E-mail: Quitsite@Roswellpark.org http://www.nysmokefree.com
North Carolina (26.4%)	July 2003	Spanish	NCI's Cancer Information Service	1-877-44U-QUIT 1-866-66-START http://www.smokefree.gov
Ohio (26.6%)	August 2003	Spanish	National Jewish Medical and Research Center	1-800-934-4840 TTY: 1-800-229-2182 http://www.standohio.org
Oklahoma (26.7%)	August 2003	Spanish, AT&T Language Line	Center for Health Promotion, Inc.	1-866-748-2436
Oregon (22.4%)	November 1998	Spanish, AT&T Language Line	Center for Health Promotion, Inc.	1-877-270-STOP (7867) TTY: 1-877-777-6534 http://www.oregonquitline.org
Pennsylvania (24.6%)	June 2002	Spanish, Telephone Translation	American Cancer Society	1-877-724-1090 TTY: 1-866-228-4327
Rhode Island (22.5%)	April 2002	Spanish, AT&T Language Line	JSI Research and Training Institute, Inc.	1-800-TRY-TO-STOP (879-8678) 1-800-8-DEJALO (833-5256) (Spanish/Portuguese) TDD: 1-800-833-1477 http://www.trytostop.org

† Compiled by Center for Tobacco Cessation, updated December 2003.
Telephone numbers and Web sites are subject to change without notice.

* Estimates of current adult smoking prevalence for each state are from the 2002 Behavioral Risk Factor Surveillance System. Centers for Disease Control and Prevention. State-specific prevalence of current cigarette smoking among adults, and policies and attitudes about secondhand smoke—United States, 2002. *Morbidity and Mortality Weekly Report* 2004;52(53):1277–1280.

†† In addition to English.

Appendix A: State Quitline Information[†]

State (Adult Smoking Prevalence*)	Date Service Began	Language Services[††]	Primary Contractor	Quitline Contact Information
South Dakota (22.6%)	January 2002	AT&T Language Line	American Cancer Society	1-866-SD-QUITS (737-8487) TTY: 1-866-228-4327
Tennessee (21.2%)	January 2001	Spanish	NCI's Cancer Information Service	1-877-44U-QUIT http://www.thestink.org
Texas (22.9%)	September 2001	Spanish, AT&T Language Line	American Cancer Society	1-877-YES-QUIT (937-7848) TTY: 1-866-228-4327
Utah (12.7%)	September 2001	Spanish	Center for Health Promotion, Inc.	1-888-567-TRUTH (8788) 1-877-2NO-FUME (266-3863) (Spanish) TDD: 1-877-777-6534 http://www.tobaccofreeutah.org
Vermont (21.2%)	February 2001	AT&T Language Line	American Cancer Society	1-877-YES-QUIT (937-7848) TTY: 1-866-228-4327 http://www.healthyvermonters.info/hi/tobacco/ tobacco.shtml
Washington (21.5%)	November 2000	AT&T Language Line	Center for Health Promotion, Inc.	1-877-270-STOP (7867) 1-877-2NO-FUME (266-3863) (Spanish) TTY: 1-877-777-6534 http://www.quitline.com
West Virginia (28.4%)	2000	Spanish	Partners In Corporate Health	1-877-966-8784 http://www.ynotquit.com
Wisconsin (23.4%)	May 2001	AT&T Language Line	Center for Health Promotion, Inc.	1-877-270-STOP (7867) 1-877-2NO-FUME (266-3863) (Spanish) TTY: 1-877-777-6534 http://www.ctri.wisc.edu/sub_dept/quit_line/out_quitline.html
Wyoming (23.7%)	October 2003	Spanish, AT&T Language Line	Mayo Clinic	1-866-WYO-QUIT TDD: 1-866-257-2971 http://wy.quitnet.com

[†] Compiled by Center for Tobacco Cessation, updated December 2003.
Telephone numbers and Web sites are subject to change without notice.

* Estimates of current adult smoking prevalence for each state are from the 2002 Behavioral Risk Factor Surveillance System. Centers for Disease Control and Prevention. State-specific prevalence of current cigarette smoking among adults, and policies and attitudes about secondhand smoke—United States, 2002. *Morbidity and Mortality Weekly Report* 2004;52(53):1277–1280.

[††] In addition to English.

Appendix B: Vendors Providing Quitline Services to States

Note: This list is intended to serve as a directory of vendors known to CDC/OSH as of December 2003 and not as an endorsement for a particular vendor.[†]

Organization	Contact Information	Web Address
American Cancer Society	1599 Clifton Road, NE Atlanta, GA 30329 Phone: 404-327-6414	http://www.cancer.org
American Lung Association	3000 Kelly Lane Springfield, IL 62707 Phone: 217-787-5864 Fax: 217-787-5916	http://www.lungusa.org
Arizona College of Public Health	P.O. Box 210482 Tucson, AZ 85721-0482 Phone: 520-318-7212 x203 Fax: 520-318-7222	http://www.nicnet.org
The Center for Health Promotion, Inc.*	12401 East Marginal Way South Tukwila, WA 98186 Phone: 206-988-7901	http://www.ghchp.com
I.Q.H. Information and Quality Healthcare	385A Highland Colony Parkway, Suite 120 Ridgeland, MS 39157 Phone: 601-957-1575 x212 Fax: 601-956-1713	http://www.iqh.org
JSI Research and Training Institute, Inc.	44 Farnsworth Street Boston, MA 02210 Phone: 617-482-9485 Fax: 617-482-0617	http://www.jsi.com
Leade Health	320 Miller Avenue, Suite E Ann Arbor, MI 48103 Phone: 734-995-0699 Fax: 734-988-1011	http://www.leadehealth.com
Mayo Clinic Tobacco Quitline	4001 NW 41st Street Rochester, MN 55901-8901 Phone: 507-538-5078 Fax: 507-538-5081	http://www.mayoclinic.com
National Jewish Medical and Research Center	1400 Jackson Street Denver, CO 80206 Phone: (303) 398-1016 Fax: 303-270-2170	http://www.nationaljewish.org
Partners in Corporate Health, Inc.*	1191 Pineview Drive, Suite F Morgantown, WV 26505 Phone: 304-599-6981 Fax: 304-599-5507	http://www.ynotquit.com

† Information subject to change without notice.
* Indicates that this vendor is a for-profit organization.

Appendix B: Vendors Providing Quitline Services to States

Note: This list is intended to serve as a directory of vendors known to CDC/OSH as of December 2003 and not as an endorsement for a particular vendor.[†]

Organization	Contact Information	Web Address
Providence Alaska Medical Center	3200 Providence Drive Anchorage, AK 99508 Phone: 907-261-4815 Fax: 907-261-6028	http://www.providence.org/alaska/default.htm
Roswell Park Cancer Institute, Department of Health Behavior	Elm & Carlton Streets Buffalo, New York 14263 Phone: 716-845-8817 Fax: 716-845-8487	http://www.roswellpark.org
University of Nevada, School of Medicine	6375 West Charleston Boulevard, Suite A100 Las Vegas, NV 89146 Phone: 1-888-866-6642 Fax: 702-877-2108	http://www.livingtobaccofree.com
University of California, San Diego, Department of Family and Preventive Medicine	9500 Gilman Drive, Mail Code 0905 La Jolla, CA 92093-0905 Phone: 858-300-1032 Fax: 858-300-1099	http://www.californiasmokershelpline.org
Wellplace (Pioneer Development and Support Services)*	7309 South 180 West Midville, UT 84047 Phone: 1-800-821-HELP	http://www.wellplace.com

[†] Information subject to change without notice.
* Indicates that this vendor is a for-profit organization.

Appendix C: Cessation Web Resources*

State Resources

State	Web Address
Arizona	www.ashline.org
California	www.californiasmokershelpline.org
Colorado	www.co.quitnet.com
Connecticut	www.ctquitline.org
Iowa	www.quitlineiowa.org
Maryland	www.smokingstopshere.com
Massachusetts	www.trytostop.org
Michigan	www.hpclearinghouse.org/tobaco/intobacco.html
New Jersey	www.nj.quitnet.com
New Mexico	www.thestink.org
New York	www.nysmokefree.com
Nevada	www.livingtobaccofree.com
Oregon	www.oregonquitline.org
Utah	www.tobaccofreeutah.org
Virginia	www.smokefreevirginia.org
Washington	www.quitline.com
West Virginia	www.ynotquit.com

Additional Resources

Organization	Web Address
American Cancer Society	www.cancer.org
Agency for Healthcare Research and Quality	www.ahrq.gov
American Legacy Foundation	www.americanlegacy.org
American Lung Association	www.lungusa.org/tobacco
Centers for Disease Control and Prevention	www.cdc.gov/tobacco/how2quit.htm
Center for Tobacco Cessation	www.ctcinfo.org
Office of the Surgeon General	www.surgeongeneral.gov/tobacco
National Cancer Institute	www.smokefree.gov
Smoke-Free Families	www.smokefreefamilies.org

* Web addresses subject to change without notice.

Appendix D: Client Education Materials Commonly Distributed by Quitlines[†*]

Organization	Title of Publication	Contact
American Cancer Society	• Set Yourself Free • Make Yours a Fresh Start Family • Living Smoke-Free for You and Your Baby • Cold, Hard Facts About Quitting • Quitting Spitting • Break Away From the Pack • Quit the Spit	1-800-227-2345 404-329-5783 http://www.cancer.org
American Legacy Foundation	• Great Start Information Packet (for pregnant and postpartum women)	1-866-66-START http://www.americanlegacy.org
American Lung Association	• Quitting for Life • Quit Smoking Action Plan • Assorted Fact Sheets	1-800-LUNG-USA http://www.lungusa.org
Centers for Disease Control and Prevention	• "I Quit!" • You Can Quit Smoking • Pathways to Freedom	1-800-311-3435 http://www.cdc.gov/tobacco
ETR (Education Training Research)	• Before You Quit Smoking • Remaining a Former Smoker • Pregnancy and Smoking • Do You Want to Be a Former Smoker? • Quit Smoking for Good: The Decide Guide • Quitting Smoking for Good: The Take Control Guide • Butts Out, Volumes 1 and 2	1-800-321-4407 http://www.etr.org
Journey Works	• Tobacco and Stress • Secondhand Smoke and Your New Baby	1-800-775-1998 http://www.journeyworks.com
National Cancer Institute	• Spit Tobacco: A Guide for Quitting	1-800-4-Cancer http://www.nci.nih.gov
New York State Smokers' Quitsite (Roswell Park)	• Break Loose: A Pack of Facts to Help You Stop Smoking Guide • Why Don't They Call Them What They Are? • Staying Tobacco-Free Guide • Various fact sheets	1-888-609-6292 http://www.nysmokefree.com

† Numbers subject to change without notice.

* This list was developed from respondents' answers to a survey on state quitlines conducted by University of California, San Diego in spring 2002. Many other materials are available and utilized by state quitlines.

Appendix E: Sample Technical Review Instrument

Instructions

Your role as a reviewer is to evaluate the proposals with regard to the proposer's ability to (1) provide services for implementation and operation of a comprehensive tobacco use quitline, as outlined in the Description of Proposal Requirements and (2) approach the Scope of Work with an understanding of what was required in the RFP. Please complete one Technical Review Instrument (score sheet) for each proposal. The instrument has been divided into separate sections with specific questions pertaining to each category. Points should be assigned in the space following the question. A space for comments is available after each section of the review instrument. Please note that some sections ask for comments on a specific issue in addition to general comments. *(Note: the comments section has been omitted from this sample in order to conserve space in this document.)* Proposals should be rated on their own merit and not compared with other proposals you are reviewing.

This scoring form may be made available to a variety of interested parties after the review process is completed, so please bear this in mind when recording your comments on this document. Confine your comments to answering the review questions directly and specifically. Avoid general comments such as *great job, looks really good*, etc. It is important that you substantiate your comments directly from the proposal, e.g., *the proposer thoroughly demonstrates the capability to address low-literacy population needs by employing methodologies....*

After the reviewers have evaluated the proposals, we will meet to review and discuss each proposal as a group. At that time, you will be asked to share comments and assessments so the review panel can select the oral presentations. The finalist oral presentations will be scored separately. To complete the process, a final discussion will be held to select the vendor for "best and final" negotiations.

I. Description of Agency's Experience with Similar Projects — **20 points**

1. Does the vendor have sufficient and appropriate experience and capability to work with governmental/nonprofit agencies? Does the vendor have experience with "800 line" operations? Does the vendor have experience with tobacco cessation counseling?
2. Does the vendor have experience collaborating with diverse health systems and provider agencies?
3. Does the vendor have sufficient expertise and experience with large agencies (e.g., state departments of health) to perform all aspects of the work?
4. Does the vendor have sufficient and appropriate capability and experience in applying appropriate telephone and data collection technology?
5. Does the vendor demonstrate sensitivity to religious, cultural, educational, and socioeconomic characteristics of potential clients?
6. Are three references provided with the following: company name; project manager/other point of contact; address; telephone; fax; e-mail address of project manager/contact; title of project/campaign; date of contract?
   ❏ YES — ❏ NO

---

† Note: Adapted from the Georgia Tobacco Use Prevention Section. The RFP developed by Georgia is available at http://www.cdc.gov/tobacco.

Appendix E: Sample Technical Review Instrument

II. Description of Organizational Capacity and Fiscal Stability	**5 points**
1. How well does this contract fit into the vendor's philosophy and/or mission? 2. Do organization chart and staff experience indicate sufficient capability to manage state quitline operations? 3. Does the vendor demonstrate sufficient fiscal, administrative, and experiential ability to manage a state government contract?	
III. Work Plan for Proposed Approach and Coordination with State Health Department	**20 points**
1. Will it be realistic to update the proposed overall work plan within the designated time frame of the implementation requirements? 2. Is each deliverable of the work plan sufficiently detailed and congruent with the program in terms of scope, duration/milestone date, and "delivery, inspection, and acceptance" criteria? 3. Are the deliverables of the work plan reasonably tied to the proposed "progress payment schedule"? 4. Are sample deliverables provided?	
IV. Proposed Funding Patterns for the Project—Costs	**15 points**
1. Does the vendor indicate a comprehensive set of program start-up costs/activities? 2. Do costs appear to be reasonable given required activity? 3. Is there sufficient explanation of budget requirements? 4. Does the vendor describe a comprehensive set of ongoing program cost components? 5. Do ongoing costs appear to be reasonable, given required activity? 6. Is there sufficient explanation of budget requirements?	
V. System Capacity and Facilities	**25 points**
1. Are indicated space requirements sufficient to reasonably accommodate required staff? 2. Is record storage capability sufficient to ensure confidentiality? 3. Is the proposed telephone system state-of-the-art, and does it include capabilities required to effectively manage call volume and overall activity (strong communication server[s], up-to-date software, automatic call distribution functionality, telephony integration)? Are the percentage of calls answered live during operating hours and average length of time to a live answer acceptable? What is the voice mail capacity? 4. Do proposed "live" response hours meet the state's needs in terms of ensuring appropriate coverage? Is there a plan for handling calls after hours and during holidays? Does the rationale for response hours indicate understanding of issues and needs of quitline? Does the vendor indicate ability to adjust for peak volume periods? 5. Is proposed monitoring system capable of collecting information required to effectively administer operations, including demographic and utilization data identifying peak hours, call volume, etc.? Does the vendor indicate ability to effectively manage operations on day-to-day and long-term basis? 6. Does the methodology for estimating call volume appear reasonable and reflect understanding of operational requirements? 7. Does the vendor demonstrate flexibility and capability to adjust as operations mature (e.g., can they handle volume expansion)?	
VI. Scientific Capacity/Service Delivery Protocol	**25 points**
1. Does the vendor describe service protocols that reflect the current science base for quitlines (e.g., PHS guidelines) and demonstrate the ability to effectively address a range of individual callers' needs? 2. Is the proposed approach comprehensive in its ability to provide appropriate motivational messages, cessation information, and referral information? 3. Does the vendor have access to a scientific advisory board? 4. Are caller follow-up protocols comprehensive, and is ongoing tracking sufficient for efficient and smooth transition to next steps? 5. Are there written procedures and policies for all aspects of operation?	
VII. Follow-Up Counseling	**15 points**
1. Does the vendor indicate follow-up service protocols that reflect current "best practices" and ability to effectively address individual callers' needs? 2. Are the scheduling and follow-up tracking methodologies reasonable and reflective of current "best practices"?	

Appendix E: Sample Technical Review Instrument

VIII. Tracking	**15 points**

1. Does the vendor indicate effective and efficient operational tracking capability? Will capability effectively provide data/information required to monitor ongoing operations and long-term outcomes?
2. Does the vendor indicate effective policies/procedures to ensure record safekeeping and confidentiality?
3. Does the vendor indicate appropriate capability for disaster management and data protection?
4. Does the vendor describe a comprehensive plan to maintain a referral resource database and capability to link referral data to geographic location of caller?
5. Are tracking procedures in compliance with HIPAA?

IX. Development of Support Material	**10 points**

1. How detailed and effective is the vendor's plan to develop and disseminate materials that address self-help techniques for both smoking and smokeless tobacco?
2. Does the vendor provide appropriate attention to the needs of low-literacy level audiences?
3. Is additional proposed support material of high quality?

X. Communication and Coordination with Statewide Media Campaign	**10 points**

1. Does the vendor propose a comprehensive approach to coordination of activities with marketing contractor, including joint planning meetings and the provision of weekly volume reports?
2. Does the vendor indicate knowledge and understanding of requirements of quitline promotional campaigns?

XI. Outreach to Referral Sources	**5 points**

1. Does the vendor propose a comprehensive and effective approach, including developing a database, to the identification and education of potential referral sources, such as public health clinics, private practitioners, etc.?
2. Does the vendor indicate commitment to assist in community education activities?

XII. Evaluation and Quality Improvement	**15 points**

1. Does the vendor propose appropriate methodologies to measure and evaluate the reach and effectiveness of ongoing project activities (e.g., quit rate/satisfaction surveys)?
2. Does the vendor have well-established procedures for tracking, analyzing, evaluating, and adjusting program components and operations, including staff performance monitoring?
3. Does the vendor propose a clear and reasonable methodology for benchmarking performance for both project management and overall evaluation purposes?
4. Does the vendor propose a comprehensive quality assurance plan?

XIII. Proposed Organization and Staffing for Project and Staff Qualifications	**20 points**

1. Does the organizational chart clearly indicate roles and responsibility of operational staff?
2. Are proposed roles, responsibilities, and staffing schedules appropriate to sufficiently service the quitline?
3. Does the vendor indicate commitment to this program by presenting qualified and highly capable staff?
4. Is the vendor assigning seasoned management to the program?
5. Are staff training procedures comprehensive and sufficient to assure up-to-date knowledge of subject matter?
6. Is there a clinical director on staff?
7. What is the staff-to-supervisor ratio?

XIV. Statement of Disclosure	**no points**

1. Does vendor hold a current or past affiliation/contractual relationship with a tobacco company?
   ❏ YES — ❏ NO
2. Does the vendor hold a current or past affiliation/contractual relationship with a tobacco-related entity, such as owners, affiliates, subsidiaries, holding companies, or companies involved in any way in the production, processing, distribution, promotion, sale, or use of tobacco?
   ❏ YES — ❏ NO

Appendix E: Sample Technical Review Instrument

Technical Review Scoring Summary Page

Reviewer number: _____   Date reviewed: _____

Proposer's name: _____

SCORES	
Description of Agency's Experience with Similar Projects	20
Description of Organizational Capacity and Fiscal Stability	5
Work Plan for Proposed Approach/Coordination with State Health Department	20
Proposed Funding Patterns—Start-up Costs	15
System Capacity and Facilities	25
Scientific Capacity/Service Delivery Protocol	25
Follow-up Counseling	15
Tracking	15
Development of Support Material	10
Communication/Coordination with Media Campaign	10
Outreach to Referral Sources	5
Evaluation/Quality Improvement	15
Proposed Organization/Project Staffing/Staff Qualifications	20
Statement of Disclosure	Y/N
Written Proposal Total Score	**200**

Summary comments: _____

_____

_____

Summary strengths and weaknesses:

_____

_____

Minor concerns that could be addressed in negotiations:

_____

_____

† Note: Adapted from the Georgia Tobacco Use Prevention Section. The RFP developed by Georgia is available at http://www.cdc.gov/tobacco.

Appendix F: Proposed Minimal Data Set for Evaluation of Telephone Cessation Helplines/Quitlines[†]

Background

The following Minimum Data Set was developed by the North American Quitline Consortium in conjunction with Canadian partners (Health Canada and the Centre for Behavioural Research in Program Evaluation, University of Waterloo). It provides a mechanism to facilitate performance monitoring, would make comparisons posssible, would be feasible, and would not impose undue burdens on quitlines. Potential funders, quitlines, scientists, vendors, and researchers have provided input to the process.

A. Recommendation for Standard Description

Quitline services are provided in many forms; for this reason, the evaluation needs to be flexible to account for the variations. When reporting on quitlines, the following elements should be described:

Minimal Descriptors
1. Overall quitline objectives (including target population).
2. Service delivery model. *A checklist could be developed to describe the types of services provided. Best-practice elements (e.g., crisis intervention protocols) should be identified and included in the above checklist.*

Additional Helpful Descriptors
1. Contextual setting (tobacco prevalence; population demographics; economic, social, and policy environment).
2. Role of quitline in comprehensive tobacco control strategy.

B. Recommendations for Minimal Data Set

The table below identifies the recommended set of indicators to be collected in a consistent manner by all quitlines. It is also recommended that both a short-term and a long-term follow-up evaluation be conducted. The short-term evaluation will help identify immediate impacts of the quitline service (particularly actions taken as a result of the quitline call), whereas the long-term follow-up evaluation will provide measures of quitline effectiveness. A 30-day and a 6-month follow-up period were recommended for the minimal data set.

Per Society for Research on Nicotine and Tobacco (SRNT) recommendations, the follow-up period is scheduled based on the *first call at which the person receives counseling.* Since quitline services vary, both the service and the time at which counseling is received by the caller should be well described so that readers can determine if comparisons across quitlines or over time can be made.

Data will be collected from three different sources:

- Administrative files.
- The intake call with those who call the quitline.
- Short- and long-term follow-up calls to evaluate service outcomes.

[†] Developed by the Centre for Behavioural Research and Program Evaluation, University of Waterloo in collaboration with the North American Quitline Consortium, with funding from Health Canada and the Canadian Cancer Society. May 2004.

Appendix F: Proposed Minimal Data Set for Evaluation of Telephone Cessation Helplines/Quitlines

INDICATORS TO BE COLLECTED AT INTAKE			
Evaluation Goal	**Indicators**	**Questions**	**Comments**
Caller Characteristics	Sex	First, I need to verify: are you male or female?	
	Age	What is your date of birth? (month, year)?	
	Pregnancy	Are you currently pregnant?	
	USA Ethnic background questions	Are you Hispanic or Latino? (yes, no, refused, don't know) Which one of these groups would you say best represents your race? 1. White 2. Black or African American 3. Asian 4. Native Hawaiian or Other Pacific Islander 5. American Indian or Alaska Native 6. Other (specify)_____ 7. Don't Know 8. Refused?	These questions are then recoded into various race/ethnicity combinations depending on one race or more being specified, etc.
	CANADIAN Ethnic background questions	To which ethnic or cultural group(s) did your ancestors belong?	Can be categorized as follows: 1. Canadian 2. English, Irish, Scottish, Welsh 3. Asian 4. Aboriginal (Native Indian, Inuit, Metis) 5. European 6. Other (specify) 7. Don't Know 8. Refused?
	Education	What is the highest level of education you have completed? (person states actual education level and interviewer categorizes)	Less than grade 9, grade 9–11 no degree, GED, high school degree, some college, college or university degree
	Health insurance	What is the name of your health insurance carrier?	Name _____ or Not insured
	Geographic region (postal/ZIP code)	What is your postal code or ZIP code?	

Appendix F: Proposed Minimal Data Set for Evaluation of Telephone Cessation Helplines/Quitlines

INDICATORS TO BE COLLECTED AT INTAKE			
Evaluation Goal	**Indicators**	**Questions**	**Comments**
Tobacco Behaviors	Tobacco use status *Series of questions to determine all forms of tobacco use*	1. Do you currently smoke cigarettes every day, some days, or not at all? 2. Do you currently use any other tobacco products? (yes, no) 3a. If yes, do you currently smoke cigars (every day, some days, not at all?) 3b. If yes—do you currently use chewing tobacco or snuff (every day, some days, not at all?)	Canada: Use national survey response options: daily, occasionally, not at all?
	Smoking intensity *Amount of tobacco smoked or chewed*	How many cigarettes do you smoke per day? How many cigars do you smoke per day? How many pouches or tins do you use per day?	These questions to follow immediately after asking if they currently use cigarettes, cigars, or chewing tobacco.
Explanatory Factors (shown to be predictive in cessation success)	Level of addiction	How soon after you wake do you smoke your first cigarette? (within first 5 min; 6 to 30 min; 31 to 60 min; more than 60 min.)	
	Self-efficacy	On a scale of 1 to 5, with 1 being not at all confident, how confident are you that you will not be smoking a year from now?	
Effectiveness of Promotion	Awareness of quitline	How did you hear about the quitline? (Media—radio, TV, newspapers Other Advertising—phone book Referrals—health professionals, workplaces, insurance)	Code all sources, but when reporting, categorize as media, other advertising and referrals.

Appendix F: Proposed Minimal Data Set for Evaluation of Telephone Cessation Helplines/Quitlines

INDICATORS TO BE COLLECTED AT FOLLOW-UP			
Evaluation Goal	**Indicators**	**Questions**	**Comments**
Service Delivery	Client satisfaction	Overall, how satisfied were you with the quitline? (very, mostly, somewhat, not at all?)	
	OPTIONAL QUESTION Extended benefit from quitline	Did you share the information you received from the quitline with anyone else? (yes, no)	
Impact Recommend 1 month grace period after FIRST call to the quitline in order for caller to complete counselling and/or set a quit date. Follow-up evaluation call to be conducted 7 months after FIRST call to quitline.			
Change in Smoking Behaviors	Tobacco use status	1. Do you currently smoke cigarettes every day, some days, or not at all? 2. Do you currently use any other tobacco products? (yes, no) 3a. If yes, do you currently smoke cigars (every day, some days, not at all?) 3b. If yes—do you currently use chewing tobacco or snuff (every day, some days, not at all?)	Canada: Use national survey response options: daily, occasionally, not at all?
	Switch from one form of tobacco to another	Use above questions regarding the types of tobacco used at intake and at follow-up.	Calculate whether switched forms of tobacco between initial call and follow-up.
	OPTIONAL Smoking intensity Determine reduction in amount smoked or chewed	How many cigarettes do you smoke per day? How many cigars do you smoke per day? How many pouches or tins do you use per day?	Reduction in amount smoked may be of interest to funders, but is not associated with health benefits nor increased success in quitting.
	Level of addiction	How soon after you wake do you smoke your first cigarette? within first 5 min; 6 to 30 min; 31 to 60 min; more than 60 min.	
Actions Taken as Result of Call			
	Quit attempts	Since you first called the quitline on (date), were you able to quit using tobacco for 24 hours or longer? (yes, no, refused, don't know)	
	OPTIONAL Length of time smoke-free	What is the longest time you went without using tobacco, even a puff or pinch?	Record in days—less than 24 hours would not qualify as a quit attempt.

Telephone Quitlines: A Resource for Development, Implementation, and Evaluation

Appendix F: Proposed Minimal Data Set for Evaluation of Telephone Cessation Helplines/Quitlines

INDICATORS TO BE COLLECTED AT FOLLOW-UP			
Evaluation Goal	Indicators	Questions	Comments
Quit Rates	7-day point prevalence	Have you smoked any cigarettes, even a puff, in the last 7 days?	
	30-day point prevalence	Have you smoked any cigarettes, even a puff, in the last 30 days?	
	6-month prolonged abstinence (allows for relapse of less than 7 days and not more than 2 weeks over 6 months). Note: Requires two questions	Since your first call to the quitline 6 months ago, was there ever a time when you smoked for 7 days in a row (7 consecutive days)? Since your first call to the quitline 6 months ago, was there ever a time when you smoked at least on the weekend for 2 weekends in a row (2 consecutive weeks)?	

INDICATORS TO BE DETERMINED FROM ADMINISTRATIVE DATA			
Evaluation Goal	Indicators	Questions	Comments
Utilization	Call volume	Total number of calls answered per (month, year).	Would be helpful to record the total number of calls, answered and unanswered.
Services Delivered	Counselling sessions delivered	Total number of callers who received at least one counselling session (reactive). Total number of callers who received more than one counselling session (proactive).	Some quitlines screen callers, then refer to a counsellor. Others provide counselling on the first call. We are interested in the number who receive counselling, not just screening.
Reach	Proportion of target population who contact the quitline	Number of individuals who contact the quitline divided by the number of [adult] smokers in the target population. Where total number in the target population is unknown, population surveys can be used.	Target population will be defined by the goals of the service (e.g., serve only smokers or smokers plus others). This should be captured by following the recommended standard description.
Costs		Most common is cost per call, including and excluding promotion costs.	Canadian investigators currently working on possible estimates of cost benefit.

Appendix G: Health Insurance Portability and Accountability Act (HIPAA)

Privacy Rule Highlights for Tobacco Quitlines

Does the Privacy Rule permit covered entity providers to disclose protected health information to a quitline without patient authorization in order to refer that patient for the quitlines services?

If a quitline is considered a health care provider under the privacy rule, a referral for treatment purposes would be permissible without patient authorization.

Does it matter whether the referral is provided by fax, phone, or otherwise?

No.

Are quitlines covered entities under the Privacy Rule?

Quitline providers may be covered entities under the Privacy Rule if they meet the definitions in the rule or are part of a larger entity that is a health care provider that conducts covered electronic transactions, a health plan, or health care clearinghouse that has not elected hybrid entity status. See the Centers for Medicare and Medicaid Services Web site decision tool for more information: http://www.cms.hhs.gov/hipaa/hipaa2/support/tools/decisionsupport/default.asp.

For the Privacy Rule requirements for covered entities, please consult the U.S. Department of Health and Human Services, Office for Civil Rights Web site at http://www.hhs.gov/ocr/hipaa.

Does the Privacy Rule preempt state laws that might apply to quitlines?

The HIPAA Privacy Rule provides a federal floor of privacy protections for individuals' individually identifiable health information where that information is held by a covered entity or by a business associate of the covered entity. State laws that are contrary to the Privacy Rule are preempted by the federal requirements, unless a specific exception applies. These exceptions include if the State law (1) relates to the privacy of individually identifiable health information and provides greater privacy protections or privacy rights with respect to such information, (2) provides for the reporting of disease or injury, child abuse, birth, or death, or for public health surveillance, investigation, or intervention, or (3) requires certain health plan reporting, such as for management or financial audits. In these circumstances, a covered entity is not required to comply with a contrary provision of the Privacy Rule.

HIPAA Web Information Sources

General Privacy Rule fact sheet:
http://www.hhs.gov/news/facts/privacy.html

Additional information on the Privacy Rule:
http://answers.hhs.gov/. Select Privacy of Health Information from the Category menu and HIPPA type in the Search Text box for specific topics, such as "referral for treatment" or "who must comply."

Appendix H

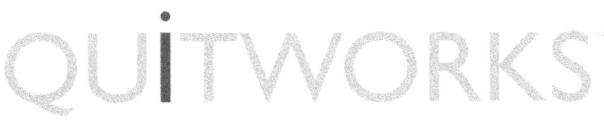

Patient stamp, label, or info. (name, record number/DOB, date)

Tobacco Treatment Enrollment
A Collaboration of the Mass. Department of Public Health & Mass. Health Plans

Tobacco Treatment Checklist

ADVISE smoker to stop: ❏ Stop-smoking advice given: "I strongly advise you to quit smoking and I to help you."

ASSESS readiness to quit: ❏ Ready to quit ❏ Thinking about quitting ❏ Not ready to quit

ASSIST smoker to quit: ❏ Brief counseling
Reasons to quit   Barriers to quitting   Lessons from past quit attempts   Set a quit date, if ready   Enlist social support

❏ Medications if appropriate
Nicotine Replacement (CIRCLE): patch gum lozenge inhaler nasal spray   Other (CIRCLE): Bupropion (Zyban/Wellbutrin SR)

ARRANGE follow-up: ❏ Refer to Try-To-STOP TOBACCO Resource Center
by faxing the lower part of this form toll-free to **1-866-560-9113**

TRY-TO-STOP TOBACCO RESOURCE CENTER OF MASSACHUSETTS
Massachusetts Resident Enrollment Form   Fax this part of form to 1-866-560-9113

PRIMARY CARE PROVIDER

primary care provider or specialist name	UPIN# (OPTIONAL)	phone (area code + number) ( )	fax (area code + number) ( )
primary care provider or specialist address		city	state	zip

PATIENT

first name	last name	date of birth (month/day/year)
phone (area code + number) ( )	May we leave a message? ❏ yes ❏ no	language preference (circle): English Spanish other (specify):	email address
patient address	city	state	zip

insurance ❏ BCBSMA ❏ BMC HealthNet Plan ❏ Fallon ❏ Harvard Pilgrim ❏ MassHealth ❏ Neighborhood Health Plan (NHP)
❏ Network Health ❏ Tufts Health Plan ❏ Other_____

The Resource Center usually calls the patient within three business days of receiving a referral. When should we call?

circle all that apply: morning   afternoon   evening   no preference

I, _____ , hereby authorize Try-To-STOP TOBACCO Resource Center of Massachusetts, (the "Resource Center"), and its representatives to disclose information about me to:
1) the American Cancer Society Quitline to the extent necessary to allow me to participate in its tobacco cessation counseling program; and
2) my primary care provider or other provider ("Provider") I designate to the Resource Center to the extent the Resource Center deems necessary to give my Provider an update of my progress in attempting to stop smoking.

I authorize NSMC to release the information on this enrollment form to the Resource Center for purposes of my participation in the QuitWorks program. I also authorize the Resource Center and its representatives to contact me upon receiving this referral from NSMC.

_____   _____
SIGNATURE OF THE PATIENT OR PATIENT'S REPRESENTATIVE   DATE

_____   _____
PRINTED NAME OF PATIENT REPRESENTATIVE   RELATIONSHIP TO PATIENT

5/03   File in chart behind Smoking Questionnaire

Copyright 2004 by the Commonwealth of Massachusetts

Appendix H

QUITWORKS

Quick Guide To Pharmacotherapy In Tobacco Treatment

NICOTINE REPLACEMENT OPTIONS

PATCHES

Nicotrol® 15 mg	Initial: MAX:	1 patch/16 hrs. Same as above	Treatment Duration: 8 wks.
* Nicoderm® CQ 21 mg 14 mg 7 mg	Initial: MAX:	1 patch/24 hrs. Same as above	Treatment Duration: 8 wks.

GUM

Nicorette® 2 mg 4 mg	Initial: MAX:	1 piece every 1–2 hrs. 24 pieces/24 hrs.	Treatment Duration: 8–12 wks.

LOZENGE

Commit® 2 mg 4 mg	1 lozenge/1–2 hrs. (wks 1–6) 1 lozenge/2–4 hrs. (wks 7–9) 1 lozenge/4–8 hrs. (wks 10–12)	Treatment Duration: 12 wks.

NASAL SPRAY

Nicotrol® NS 10 mg/ml	Initial: MAX:	1–2 doses/hr. 5 doses/hr. or 40 doses/day	Treatment Duration: 3–6 mos.

INHALER

Nicotrol® Inhaler 10 mg/cartridge	Initial: MAX:	6–16 cartridges/day 16 cartridges/day	Treatment Duration: 3–6 mos.

NON-NICOTINE MEDICATION

BUPROPION HCL SR

* Zyban® 150 mg tablets	Initial: MAX:	150 mg/day (days 1–3) 300 mg/day (day 4+) 300 mg/day	Treatment Duration: 7–12 wks.

Inclusion of this adult dosage chart is strictly for the convenience of the prescribing provider. Please consult the Physicians' Desk Reference for complete product information and contraindications. This chart does not indicate or authorize insurance benefit coverage for any of these medications. For insurance benefit information, the patient will need to contact his/her insurer directly. The cost or provision of these medications is not included as any part of the Try-To-STOP TOBACCO Resource Center of Massachusetts or QuitWorks program.

* NORMALLY AVAILABLE FROM HOSPITAL PHARMACY

Make smoking history.

Copyright 2004 by the Commonwealth of Massachusetts

Appendix I

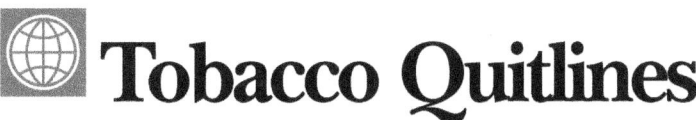

Tobacco Quitlines
at a glance

What are tobacco quitlines?

Quitlines are telephone-based tobacco cessation services. Since the late 1980's, quitlines have been established in many countries, states and provinces. Most are accessed through a toll-free telephone number and provide a combination of services including educational materials, referral to local programs, and individualized telephone counseling. Counselors answer callers' questions about the cessation process and help them develop an effective plan for quitting.

Reactive quitlines only respond to incoming calls. Proactive quitlines handle incoming calls and also follow up the initial contact with additional outbound calls, to help initiate a quit attempt or to help prevent relapse. In some cases, as when smokers give consent in their doctors' offices to be called by a counselor, the contact is entirely proactive. Proactive telephone counseling has been shown to have a marked effect on callers' probability of success in quitting and in maintaining long-term abstinence from tobacco use, comparable to the effects of pharmacotherapies.

Where are they available?

Brazil, Iran, New Zealand, South Africa, many European countries, some countries in Asia, and most Australian, Canadian, and U.S. states and provinces have publicly financed quitlines. Some employers and private health insurers provide quitlines for their employees and members. Many new quitlines have been set up in recent years, as evidence of their efficacy has become more solid and as tobacco control programs worldwide have become more common. Quitlines vary greatly in scale and sophistication.

Why have quitlines become popular?

Easy access. Traditionally, tobacco users have faced various barriers in accessing cessation services, including:
- Sporadic availability, geographically and over time
- Transportation difficulties
- Childcare responsibilities
- Financial cost of participating.

Quitlines reduce these barriers by allowing users to access service from their own homes at a time that is convenient for them, and usually at no cost to themselves. Partly for these reasons, surveys have shown that tobacco users are much more likely to use telephone-based services than face-to-face programs.

Benefits of centralization. Because it provides services over the telephone, a quitline can serve a large geographic

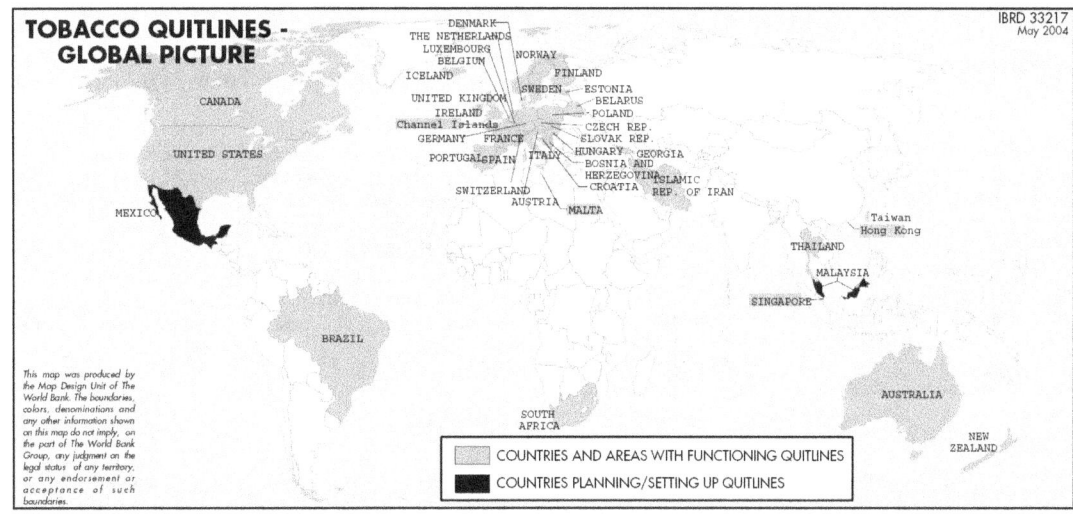

May 2004

This fact sheet was developed and prepared by the World Bank; used with permission.

Appendix I

area from a single, centralized base of operations. So unlike traditional cessation programs in which it is common for participants to have to wait until a group forms, quitlines are able to operate year-round, often with extended hours of business and multilingual capabilities.

The benefits of centralization include:
- Economies of scale, leading to more efficient utilization of counseling resources
- Standardized training
- Better quality control
- Ease of evaluation.

Ease of promotion. Most comprehensive tobacco control programs include a media component designed to counteract the effects of tobacco industry advertising. This key part of successful anti-tobacco programs can be very costly, necessitating prudent spending decisions. Media programs are a convenient way to promote cessation services, since advertisements can carry a single telephone number and air across a wide area. This is more efficient than promoting an array of local programs, each with its own method of accessing service. And quitlines can refer callers to local programs as appropriate, thus serving both as a direct cessation service provider and as a hub of coordinated services.

Strong evidence of quitline efficacy

Reactive quitlines: Two studies support use of a reactive quitline in the context of a comprehensive tobacco control program. A California study found that a well-promoted quitline providing a single comprehensive counseling session of about 50 minutes increased quit attempts and reduced relapse, relative to an intervention of self-help materials alone (Zhu et al. 1996). Counties in New York State where a quitline was promoted had significantly higher quit rates than those without such promotion, even though the majority of evaluated quitters did not access the service, indicating that quitline promotion in itself may increase cessation on a population level (Ossip-Klein et al. 1991).

Proactive quitlines: The evidence for proactive quitlines is more thorough. Several meta-analytical reviews have established that proactive telephone counseling is an effective intervention for smoking cessation (Lichtenstein et al. 1996, Fiore et al. 2000, Hopkins et al. 2001, Stead et al. 2004). The most recent of these examined 13 studies of proactive interventions and found that callers who received counseling were successful at least 50% more often than those who only received self-help materials (odds ratio of 1.56) (Stead et al. 2004). The *U.S. Public Health Clinical Practice Guideline* and the *Guide to Community Preventive Services* recommend proactive quitlines as a way to help smokers quit (Fiore et al. 2000, Hopkins et al. 2001).

A large randomized, controlled trial (n=3,030) that served as the basis for the California Smokers' Helpline, the first publicly supported, statewide quitline, found that telephone counseling increased the percentage of smokers making a quit attempt and decreased the rate of relapse for those attempts, and found a strong dose-response relationship between the level of intended treatment intensity (i.e., number of follow-up sessions) and the treatment effect (Zhu et al. 1996).

Further research has demonstrated the continued effectiveness of the California quitline after it scaled up to statewide operation (Zhu et al. 2002). Borland et al. (2001) found similar results for a quitline service in Victoria, Australia. These studies increase confidence that the efficacy found in clinical trials can carry over to "real world" settings. With the efficiencies inherent in centralized, telephone-based operations, quitlines appear to be a cost-effective way to deliver cessation assistance (McAlister et al. 2004).

Quitlines as part of comprehensive tobacco control programs

Most quitlines are supported by state or national health agencies, through tobacco taxes or other public funds. They are often the government's chief or only contribution to providing direct tobacco cessation services, with the rest of its tobacco control funding earmarked for other efforts such as educating people about the harm caused by tobacco use, preventing initiation of tobacco use among young people, and reducing exposure to second hand smoke. If resources were not available to make progress in these areas, it is doubtful that a quitline alone would be a worthwhile investment of public health funds. But in the context of comprehensive tobacco control efforts, a quitline can help to advance larger goals of the program, such as normalizing cessation and eliminating disparities in tobacco use or access to treatment.

Practical considerations

The range of services provided: Quitline callers have a wide range of expectations, so most well established quitlines offer a wide range of services. Adult smokers wanting help to quit are the most common callers, but there are also those who are not yet ready to quit, or who have already quit. There are smokers of cigarettes, cigars, and pipes, and callers who use chewing tobacco or other smokeless tobacco. There are callers of all ages, including minors, and callers who speak different languages. In all of these categories, some want counseling; others just want printed information or referral. Some callers have particular needs such as learning more about smoking while pregnant, or quitting tobacco while managing a psychological condition such as bipolar disorder or schizophrenia. There are non-tobacco-users calling on behalf of friends and family members, and health care professionals or others trying to decide whether to refer their patients, students, or neighbors. Comprehensive quitlines develop protocols, resources, and staff training for each situation.

Evidence-based structured protocols guide the flow of counseling sessions and remind counselors of topics considered to affect quitting success. Counselors using clinically validated protocols help clients to:

This fact sheet was developed and prepared by the World Bank; used with permission.

- Clarify and enhance their motivation to quit
- Boost their self-efficacy for quitting
- Identify situations that will trigger an urge to use tobacco, and plan effective strategies for getting through them without tobacco
- Identify ways to get the social support they need
- Commit to a quit date, often with counselor follow-up for accountability and extra support.

Staffing: Quitlines are staffed to meet demand, which is largely determined by the intensity and timing of promotion. Rather than staying open around the clock, most quitlines focus their resources on peak daytime and evening hours. The staffing plan must take into account both the overall demand for service over time, and the demand at any given moment, especially during the "bursts" of calls that occur when mass media advertisements are aired. For new quitlines, the number of staff required may be calculated by estimating the likely number of callers, which in turn may be done by comparing the promotional plan with similar campaigns elsewhere. Most quitlines require between 30 minutes and two hours of counselor time per caller, depending on the intensity and number of counseling sessions provided. Maintaining a balance between counselors' productivity and their availability for incoming calls is one of the main challenges of quitline operations, but one which becomes more manageable as the scale grows.

When recruiting counselors, it is helpful to keep in mind that most of the evidence for the efficacy of quitlines is based on the work of paraprofessional counselors using structured protocols, indicating that postgraduate education and licensure are not necessary. Instead of graduate training, most quitlines look for candidates with natural counseling skills such as empathy, reflective listening, and the ability to guide clients through a structured problem-solving process. These skills are crucial to quitline quality and effectiveness.

Training and supervision: A quitline's training program is another key to assuring quality in its services. At a minimum, a good training program addresses:

- The psychology of tobacco use and the process of habit formation, maintenance, and extinction
- General principles of counseling and motivational interviewing
- Effective counseling techniques for behavior modification
- Challenging counseling scenarios, such as crisis calls and callers with psychiatric issues
- Multicultural counseling
- Effective case management practices, including use of protocols
- Health issues related to tobacco use and cessation
- NRT and other quitting aids.

Following up the initial training with a regular program of continuing education helps counselors continuously develop their skills and ensures that their knowledge of the field is up to date.

Besides providing training, quitline supervisors and managers oversee coverage of incoming calls, effective case management, and productivity. They monitor and debrief sessions and make sure the services provided are helpful, appropriate, and factually accurate. They also ensure the program's compliance with applicable laws and ethical guidelines governing the provision of telephone counseling.

Evaluation: Successful and sustainable quitline operation requires rigorous evaluation. Baseline data include, at a minimum, how callers heard about the quitline, demographic variables such as age, ethnicity, and education, type of tobacco used and level of consumption. Process data include percentage of calls answered live and number of callers (especially members of target populations) receiving each type of service. Follow-up data include quit status, length of abstinence, and satisfaction with quitline services. For quitlines serving large numbers of callers, following up a randomly selected sample is adequate.

It may not be feasible or even desirable for every quitline to conduct its own clinical trial to ensure efficacy, but all quitline funding should include an allocation for program evaluation to address key questions:

- What contribution is the quitline making to the overall tobacco control program?
- Is it successful in reaching target populations, especially high-risk and underserved groups?
- Are callers satisfied with services received?
- What percentages of callers make a quit attempt, and maintain abstinence (e.g., for 6 months)?
- Are the results comparable to other published outcomes?

It is important when citing results to identify clearly any characteristics of the population that received service that may have had a bearing on their success, and to address whether and why any participants were excluded from the analysis.

Promotion: Increasing public awareness of quitline services can be done in various ways. Mass media advertising—television, radio, newspapers, billboards, and other media—usually plays a central role in promotion. Successful mass media campaigns identify their target audience and do thorough marketing research before launching ads. Cultural and linguistic appropriateness is especially important. Low-cost promotional strategies have been successfully used in some countries, such as requiring manufacturers to print the quitline telephone number on cigarette packages.

Health care providers are natural partners for quitlines and can play a major role in increasing their utilization. Providers who ask all patients whether they use tobacco, advise quitting, and refer patients to quitlines for comprehensive cessation counseling can have a profound impact on patient health. Therefore many quitlines make special efforts to build linkages with health care providers. As with mass media advertising, promoting quitlines through health care systems not only generates calls and

This fact sheet was developed and prepared by the World Bank; used with permission.

Appendix I

helps callers quit, but also increases cessation among people who do not call the quitline.

Technology: A robust and scalable telephone system greatly facilitates operations by allowing quitlines to:

- Queue calls and route them to counselors according to pre-established priorities
- Monitor calls
- Track and report on performance (e.g., percentage of calls answered live)
- Expand capacity as needed.

Information systems are very important to the smooth functioning of proactive quitlines, which over time may serve hundreds of thousands of callers, each receiving service spread out over several calls, in some cases with different counselors. Computer networks and databases must be able to store sufficient information on all contacts with individual callers to ensure a seamless delivery of services. Integration of the communication and information systems, using off-the-shelf Computer Telephony Integration (CTI) software, can greatly enhance efficiency. Other technologies have the potential to expand the range of services offered. Interactive Voice Response (IVR) systems, for example, allow callers to access personalized automated messages based on information they provide. Other emerging options include web-based interfaces, integration with email, and sending text messages or even images and short films to cell phone users.

Costs: The costs of establishing and running a quitline can vary widely. Communications and information systems can be a significant start-up cost, although fairly inexpensive options with limited functionality are available. The two largest ongoing expenses are usually for promotion and staffing. The U.S. Centers for Disease Control and Prevention recommend that new quitlines spend as much money on promotion in the first couple of years as on all other direct costs combined. (Quitline promotion, it should be remembered, not only generates calls to the quitline but also promotes cessation in the general population.) Over time, the cost for promotion may stabilize or even decrease as the quitline builds referral relationships with organizations and individuals in the community. Staffing costs, on the other hand, tend to increase steadily over the years.

Steps in setting up a quitline

- Assess the need for cessation services in the population, considering the prevalence of tobacco use in various communities and their readiness to respond to cessation messaging.
- Determine how direct provision of service fits into the overall plan for decreasing tobacco use in the population.
- Identify a reliable funding source and determine a funding level appropriate to the quitline's intended role in the overall tobacco control program. Tobacco taxes, where available, are a commonly used resource for quitlines.
- Determine a budget and strategies for promotion. Promotional budgets that are roughly equivalent to operational budgets are common.
- Create a competitive process to select a quitline operator. A Request for Proposals (RFP) process, in which the funding agency provides a thorough description of the quitline services to be provided and invites proposals from interested parties, is common.
- Create a similar process for selecting a media contractor. Require both contractors to coordinate their activities with each other.
- Write contracts with the selected providers that include firm deadlines for delivery of service.
- Closely monitor the contracts to ensure adherence to standards and deadlines. Perform ongoing evaluation to ensure the quitline's effectiveness and continued relevance to the overall tobacco control program.

Careful planning, an adequate budget, and rigorous evaluation will help ensure a successful quitline.

Key Resources for More Information

Anderson CM, Zhu SH. *The California Smokers' Helpline: A Case Study*. Sacramento, CA: California Department of Health Services; May 2000.

Borland R, Segan CJ, Livingston PM, Owen N. The effectiveness of callback counselling for smoking cessation: a randomized trial. *Addiction*. 2001;96:881-889.

Centers for Disease Control and Prevention. *Quitline Resource Guide: Strategies for Effective Development, Implementation, and Evaluation*. Atlanta: U.S. Department of Health and Human Services, Centers for Disease Control and Prevention, National Center for Chronic Disease Prevention and Health Promotion, Office on Smoking and Health, 2004.

European Network of Quitlines: Guide to Best Practice. Available at www.enqonline.org.

Lichtenstein E, Glasgow RE, Lando HA, Ossip-Klein DJ, Boles SM. Telephone counseling for smoking cessation: rationales and meta-analytic review of evidence. *Health Education Research: Theory and Practice* 1996;1:243-257.

Stead LF, Lancaster T, Perera R. Telephone counselling for smoking cessation (Cochrane Review). In: *The Cochrane Library* Issue 2, 2004. Chichester, UK: John Wiley & Sons, Ltd.

Zhu SH, Anderson CM, Tedeschi GT, Rosbrook B, Johnson CE, Byrd M, Gutiérrez-Terrell E. Evidence of real-world effectiveness of a telephone quitline for smokers. *New England Journal of Medicine* 2002;347(14):1087-1093.

Zhu SH, Stretch V, Balabanis M, Rosbrook B, Sadler G, Pierce JP. Telephone counseling for smoking cessation: effects of single-session and multiple-session intervention. *Journal of Consulting and Clinical Psychology* 1996;64:202-211.

This fact sheet was developed and prepared by the World Bank; used with permission.

www.ingramcontent.com/pod-product-compliance
Lightning Source LLC
Chambersburg PA
CBHW081726170526
45167CB00009B/3718